You Shall Say To

THIS MOUNTAIN,

'Move From Here To There.'

A Pastor and Medical Doctor defines faith as taught
by Jesus and displayed by the Centurion, then gives
insight into mechanisms of disease to identify the
specific mountain that needs to be moved.

By Greg Berglund, M.D., M.Div.

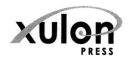
Xulon
PRESS

Table of Contents

USE YOUR AUTHORITY

Dedication

To Patty, my beloved wife
and devoted mother of our children:
Kalley, Rose, Anne, and Tom.

Acknowledgements

Special thanks to those in our small fellowship group who share their gifts, encouragement, and prayers. Thanks also to those participating in *Healing on the Hill*, a healing ministry at North Heights Lutheran Church. Thanks also to those God used to disciple and equip me for the works of ministry including the members of the outreach group called *Living Power*, a Pastor at Daystar Ministries in Fargo, North Dakota who prayed for me to receive the baptism of the Holy Spirit, Pastor Arthur Grimstad for his solid biblical teachings, Pastor Morris Vaagenes at North Heights Church who released me into many opportunities for ministry, and to the healing ministries of various ones whose books and examples contributed to my training in doing the works of the kingdom of God.

I am also grateful for the many teachers, medical doctors, and other professionals that contributed to my medical education. I studied medicine at a secular school, the University of North Dakota School of Medicine. As we were taught about the incredible functions and features of human anatomy and physiology, I repeatedly heard professors stating that God made us this way.

The information in this book regarding various diseases is very basic and superficial and regarded as common knowledge. This book attempts to identify the cause of the disease states so as to understand how to speak to THIS MOUNTAIN. For this purpose I frequently referenced a textbook of pathology, *The Pathologic Basis of Disease*, 5th edition, by Robbins et al.

All gratitude goes to God the Father, Jesus Christ His Son, and the Holy Spirit who work in us salvation, sanctification, empowerings, and gifts for His glory and the work of the ministry.

Introduction

My father repeatedly stressed the importance of authority. He never said to me, "Authority is important," or "Obedience to authority is expected." He did say occasionally, as I went off to school, "If your teacher tells you to do something, you be sure to do it." I remember him saying as I engaged in sports, "If your coach tells you what to do, make sure that you do what he says." If I brought him a question about something that happened at school, he listened to me, but invariably looked for and sided with the teacher's position on the issue.

He was teaching me obedience to authority. As I look back on it, I realize this was perhaps the most important lesson for me to learn. My father did not explain why he gently insisted on obedience to authority. I never had a discussion with him about the reasons why he stressed this; though I am sure he had good reasons. He knew that no teacher or coach is perfect. Still he defaulted to the teacher's and coach's authority without qualification. What he was telling me to do was consistent with how he lived. I do not have any remembrance of him breaking any laws or disregarding or despising authority.

My father was teaching me about faith. He would not have described obedience to authority as a process for learning faith. He did not understand that he was establishing faith in me. I am sure that he did understand the benefits of obedience to authority for purposes of protection and provision. I believe he knew that what he was insisting on would be for my benefit. He knew that such obedience would not always be easy or convenient. Like any father's hopes for his children, he wanted me to succeed in school, work, relationships, and life in general.

Without knowing it, he was teaching me about faith. Faith is understanding authority, being under authority, and being in authority. Most do not define faith in this way. Careful study of the Word of God uncovers this profound truth about faith. Authority and faith are closely linked. Discovery of this understanding of faith is paramount to understanding the mustard seed faith about which Jesus spoke.

Most Christian believers desire an increase in faith. The apostles who followed Jesus on earth saw the importance of faith so they asked Jesus to increase their faith. Jesus answered with a discussion about a mustard seed faith that can move mountains. How do we understand and employ this faith? How can we have our faith increased just as the apostles did?

Since becoming a Spirit-filled Christian, I have had an interest in praying for healing, but I rarely saw results until I learned some very important truths from the Word of God which are unpacked in this book. I will attempt to show believers how to increase your faith for healing and miracles and bring healing to diseases and infirmities. Specifically, we will look at the particular faith that the Centurion understood — the great faith that Jesus had not seen the likes of in all Israel. I will also provide some specific information regarding various categories of diseases and their mechanisms of action so that you can speak specifically to "THIS MOUNTAIN."

Throughout my primary education years I was mostly interested and engaged in the sciences and math. I always thought that my career would involve these disciplines. I went through a personal awakening in my faith in my college years and sensed a call to become a Pastor, but I never lost my love for the sciences. After working as a Pastor for a dozen years, I went back to school to become a medical doctor. not to leave ministry but add to it. As I went through medical school and learned about the mechanisms of various diseases, I was mindful of these words from Jesus about speaking to "THIS MOUNTAIN."

If you are going to minister to someone who had back pain, how would you speak to that mountain? If you were to minister to someone who had Crohn's disease, how would you direct that ministry? What would you say and do to someone who has recurrent migraine headaches? How can you use mustard seed faith to attend to matters in your own life, your family, your work, and your relationships?

Section 1

WHAT IS FAITH?

———————◆———————

This book is arranged in four sections: 1) What is Faith; 2) Know Your Authority; 3) Mechanisms of Disease; and 4) Use Your Authority. This first section establishes a definition of faith as taught by Jesus. This same faith was present in the Centurion who came to Jesus seeking healing for his paralyzed servant. Jesus marveled at the Centurion's faith, saying that He had not seen anyone in all of Israel with such great faith.

Jesus taught the apostles about this kind of faith. This first section lays a foundation for a faith that can address THIS MOUNTAIN, telling it to move from here to there.

Chapter 1

Mustard Seed Faith

The home I live in gets water from a well. A few years ago we began to notice some silt in the bathtub and the sink. We consulted a water expert who looked at what was happening. He stated it was likely oxidized manganese precipitating out of the water. So I installed a separate unit to remove iron, sulfur, and manganese. This helped briefly, but soon the same sediment was present. A little later fine brown sand began to appear in the sinks and tubs. Then I installed a small filter to collect this sand, but soon this filter was overwhelmed.

Then I did something that every Christian should do in this type of situation. I stood over the access to the well in my front yard and said, "In the name of Jesus, I command this well to stop sending sand into my water supply." From that moment on and for the next six months there was no longer any sand or silt coming into our water supply to our house. Glory to God.

Jesus said, "If you have faith as a grain of mustard seed, you will say to this mountain, 'move from here to there,' and it will move; and nothing will be impossible for you" Matthew 17:20. Certainly the amount of sand present in our water supply was no mountain, but it did respond to my words of command in the name of Jesus. For the next six months our water was clear. To complete the story, we then began having large amounts of sand in our home's water supply. We eventually had to replace the casing of the well which was breaking down.

Faith and Authority

All of us have seemingly immovable situations in our lives. When you believe in Jesus you are given authority by Him over certain things—but not everything. The Centurion, whose servant was at home dying, understood the authority that Jesus had. This Centurion also understood his own position where he was placed in the army. The authority that he was given in the army and whose authority he was under was clear and well defined. Jesus said this man had great faith. We do not often define faith in the way that Jesus did. I would have said to the Centurion that he has a good understanding of his position in the army's chain of command. Jesus called this great faith. This gives us a big clue about the workings of faith that Jesus and His disciples operated in, providing a huge insight into the victorious faith that overcomes the world and is more precious than gold.

Most Christians do not understand the authority that they have been given in Christ. Of the ones who do understand it, most of them do not use it. Of the ones who know and use their authority in Christ, some of them are misusing it or demonstrating it with certain methodologies and attitudes that may be ineffective or may turn other people away.

Speak to This Mountain

What did Jesus intend when He instructed His disciples about faith? He spoke about a mountain moving from here to there. How do we understand this teaching? How do we make application of this to our daily lives? Jesus instructed His disciples about how to employ this faith in God. The disciples understood these truths and put them to use. They returned to Jesus rejoicing at the power of God at work through their own words and actions. They saw people healed of diseases and delivered from the power of the devil. We also can understand and act using this same mustard seed faith.

Faith speaks. Faith enables a Christian to speak to a mountain. "If you have faith..., you will SAY to this mountain..." Mustard seed faith is a faith that speaks. Faith is active, engaging its object with words. Words coming from one with faith have great power – even to move mountains. Faith speaks to THIS mountain, addressing a specific mountain — not just any mountain. This faith does not speak to all mountains at once, so as to give any one of them permission to move. "If you have faith..., you will say to THIS mountain..."

The Gift of Faith

Jesus brings forgiveness of sins, healing of diseases, and deliverance from the enemy. We participate in and appropriate these provisions by hearing the Word of God and believing those words. The people of the Christian church generally have lots of faith for forgiveness of sins. We believe that if you confess and repent, God will be faithful to forgive your sins. We do not have that same faith and confidence for healings, signs, and wonders. The same name of Jesus accomplishes all of this. The apostles saw Jesus' authority to perform miracles and heal the sick, so they asked Jesus for increased faith. This gift of faith can be learned and understood. Jesus taught this mustard seed faith to His disciples. The Word of God records this teaching, making it available for us to grow in faith and begin to see God's Kingdom and authority advance in our midst with miracles and healings to the glory of God.

This was a normal practice of the early church for several centuries, but it has dwindled in most developed societies today. Many Christians believe that God might heal only on rare occasions, or attribute healing from God as occurring only through medical strategies and procedures. Many people pray for healing with little or no results. However, throughout the world there are abundant testimonies of miracles and healings, especially in developing countries. Some conclude that the outpouring of the Spirit of God for signs and wonders is unlike any other time.

The Great Commission

Jesus went about the region, preaching the gospel, teaching in the synagogues, and healing diseases.[1] Then He taught His disciples to do the same things and sent them out. At the end of his ministry He told His disciples the great commission.

> "And Jesus came and said to them, 'All authority in heaven and on earth has been given to me. Go therefore and make disciples of all nations, baptizing them in the name of the Father and of the Son and of the Holy Spirit, teaching them to observe all that I have commanded you...'" Matthew 28:18-20.

What did Jesus teach them to observe and command them to do? He taught them to go, preach, teach, and heal. These are the same things that Jesus did. Disciples of Jesus are to teach and disciple others to do these things, including healing. Healing does not seem to happen so much in most churches because it is not taught. Few people know how to release this power of God that dwells in believers. What I will show you in the Scriptures is very simple and obvious, yet rarely practiced among believers. Those who practice and do the words of the Scriptures experience life transforming ministry. This transformation occurs in the one ministering and the one receiving ministry.

> "For the eyes of the Lord run to and fro throughout the whole earth, to show his might on behalf of those whose heart is blameless toward him" 2 Chronicles 16:9.

There are people with illnesses, sicknesses, and all manner of pains all around us. There are abundant opportunities for ministry. Having some training and employment in the various fields of medicine gives all the more connections to people needing help, but to minister the good news of the gospel does not require medical training. You do not need any background or training in medicine, physiology, or anatomy to minister healing to another person in the name of Jesus. There are things that you do need and strategies that you can learn in order to begin to see growth and results in healing ministry.

The practice of medicine can inform ministry and ministry can occur through medicine. A profession in medicine presents opportunities for ministry. Christians can benefit from reasonable evidence coming from research and the scientific method. In James 3:17 we read: "But the wisdom from above is pure, then peaceable, gentle, and open to reason." Research and scientific methodology use reason and observation to gather truths. This knowledge must always be subject to the eternal truth of the Word of God.

Revelation

The truth of the Scriptures is hidden from the wise and learned, but revealed by the Holy Spirit to anyone who calls on Him and humbles himself before the Lord God and His Word. Proper understanding of God's Word requires this revelation that comes from the Holy Spirit. In John 7:17, Jesus states that if anyone DOES what the Word of God says, he will find that these words are true. We often think that we acquire knowledge by mental exercise. Jesus states that we acquire awareness of the truth of Scripture by doing those words. We might prefer to try to do something after we have understood it and studied it, but the Scriptures state the opposite. The words of Jesus state that understanding comes by doing the Word. The Scriptures say we gain understanding by doing God's will and by revelation of the Holy Spirit.

I am not at all against classroom learning and study strategies. I did go to 29 years of school. A person who reads and learns everything there is to know about pole vaulting is not a pole vaulter until taking the pole in his hands and practicing his technique. A person who knows a lot about cars is not authorized to drive legally until demonstrating satisfactory skills in the behind the wheel driver's test. In the sport of baseball, homerun leaders are often strikeout leaders. They keep trying and do not lose heart, believing that they can accomplish something productive each time at the batter's plate. A Christian who wishes to minister healing to others must also learn to speak to "this mountain." Sometimes it feels like you are stepping out of the boat to walk on water toward Jesus, but if you minister to others with a humble attitude and truly care for them, they will be blessed no matter what may or may not occur.

Chapter 2

Saved, Assured, and Filled

Too often we skip over basic essentials of being a Christian. One who reads this book or attends a church is not thereby automatically established as a Christian. If one stands in a garden, this does not make him a flower. If one is in a garage, he is not automatically an automobile. To be a Christian, we must understand and receive from the Word of God the good news of the gospel of Jesus Christ. We live in a Judeo-Christian society which has defined Christianity rather than Christianity defining the culture. We must have a biblical look at our culture, not a cultural view of the Bible. This chapter is devoted to these basic essentials of faith.

Saved

A Christian accepts Jesus as Lord and Savior, has received forgiveness of sins, and places trust in Him for salvation and eternal life. A Christian has invited Jesus into his or her heart and yields to Him as Lord. More important than any works or deeds we do, believers are to rejoice in that they are saved and have their names written in the book of life. Actually we are not able to do any works that matter for eternity unless we know Him and follow in the good works that He arranged beforehand that we should walk in them.[1]

How can you become a Christian, receive salvation, and receive the gift of eternal life with our Heavenly Father? Will good behavior and doing charitable acts somehow place you in favor with God? No amount of good deeds or efforts will pay the penalty for our sins. If someone keeps the whole law but fails in just one point, he is nevertheless guilty of breaking the law.[2] Sin carries a penalty of death; death is required of those who sin. All of us have sinned and fall short of God's holiness and glory. All people are under the penalty of death and cannot stand on our own before God and His holiness.

This is an eternal law, a forever truth, governing all of creation and all time. This is true even before creation and time existed. God holiness and righteousness does not tolerate sin. When Lucifer rebelled, God drove him out of heaven. There is no possibility of redemption for Lucifer and the angels who followed him in their rebellion against God. For humans, there is a possibility for redemption, but payment for sin requires the shedding of blood. Before Jesus came to earth, God allowed a substitutionary sacrifice to suffice in paying the penalty. The shedding of blood from sacrificed animals temporarily paid for or atoned for human sin.

Then God's Son, Jesus, as God himself, a sacrificial lamb without sin, paid the penalty for sin once and for all people and all time. Jesus' death and resurrection has retroactive and proleptic effects, that is to say, that one time event in the span of history worked backward and forward to provide a way for all sinners to be restored in relationship with God the Father. The whole of Scripture is about a Father who lost His children and has gone to great lengths to get them back. Jesus is the way to the Father. He is not the destination; the Father is the destination. Jesus is the way by which sinners can return to the life giving relationship with God the Father.

Those who believe in Jesus and receive Him into their hearts and lives are made clean by His shedding of blood and by His death. He who was without sin became sin for us to set us free from this penalty and bring us to relationship with His Father in heaven. So Jesus is the only way to the Father because He is the only sinless human whose death could satisfy this penalty required by God. God does not accept any other way for sinners to return to Him because the penalty has already been paid by Jesus. He will not accept another way because it was a great sacrifice to send His only beloved Son to die for us. To allow any other way to God would diminish this great sacrifice.

Furthermore, any other way does not pay the penalty for sin, because no other has lived sinless and taken our sins upon themselves.

The free gift of forgiveness, redemption, and restoration to the Father is available to anyone who believes in Jesus and places trust in Him for payment of the penalties for sin. No sin or situation exceeds God's grace. All can come confidently before His throne of grace to receive forgiveness and redemption. However, human pride wants to attempt to make things right ourselves, to correct the wrongs and hopefully show ourselves acceptable to God. This was never God's plan; it is never successful. The only answer for the human problem is death. Any Christian counseling not built upon this solution for the human problem opposes the work of Jesus on the cross. God's plan was never to fix the human problem, but to crucify it, then give newness of life through His Son.

Identification

Paul said he was crucified with Christ and lived then by faith in the Son of God.[3] Not only did Jesus die on the cross FOR our sins, we who believe died WITH Him. This identification with Christ's death is essential for living by faith in the Son of God. Many believers understand that Jesus Christ died FOR their sins to bring us back to the Father. Not so many understand this identification WITH Christ's death. Not so many live as ones crucified WITH Christ. Believers were crucified WITH Christ on the cross; we died WITH Him. This accomplishes God's demand for righteousness, satisfies the payment of the penalty of death, and empowers our lives now lived in the flesh by faith in the Son of God.

> "You were buried *with* him in baptism, in which you were also raised *with* him through faith in the working of God, who raised him from the dead" Colossians 2:12 (italics mine).

> "If *with* Christ you died to the elemental spirits of the universe, why do you live as if you still belonged to the world?" Colossians 2:20 (italics mine).

"For you have died, and your life is hid *with* Christ in God" Colossians 3:3 (italics mine).

Jesus will not force His will upon you. He waits for you to respond to what He has accomplished for you. He waits for your invitation, standing at the door of your heart and knocking, hoping you will open the door for Him to enter into your heart. If you believe this good news of the gospel of Jesus Christ and accept Him and your Savior and Lord, then from your heart you can pray this prayer for your salvation:

> Father in heaven, I come to you in the name of your Son Jesus. I am a sinner in need of a Savior. I repent of my sins and ask you to forgive me of all of my sins. I trust you to cleanse me from where I have offended you and others. I thank you that you sent your Son Jesus to pay the penalty I deserve. I ask you, Jesus, to come into my heart and life to be my Lord and Savior. I open my heart, soul, mind, and body to welcome you. I ask you to bring me to your Father and grant me eternal life. I thank you that you are faithful to your word. I thank you that you died for me and that I died with you on the cross. I thank you for salvation and eternal life. I pray this in the name of Jesus Christ. Amen.

Assurance of Salvation

Furthermore, we can be assured of our salvation. More than just hoping in eternal life, this assurance is a confidence based on God's Word, faith in that Word, and the witness of the Holy Spirit to our inner being. In 1 John 5:13 we read: "I write to you who believe in the name of the Son of God, that you might *know* that you have eternal life" (italics mine).

How can we know with certainty that we are forgiven of sins and have eternal life? Our own reasoning or philosophies cannot generate such assurance. Our emotions or experiences cannot provide this confidence. We also cannot will ourselves to know this truth with certainty. No amount of good deeds can manufacture this assurance; nor can it be obtained by avoiding all sinful behavior. Rather, it is solely a gift from God to the inner being of a believer. It stands in Romans 8:16, "it is the Spirit himself bearing witness with our spirit that we are children of God."

Yet there are some ways by which we position ourselves to receive this gift of the Holy Spirit. James 4:8 says "Draw near to God, and He will draw near to you." We can initiate drawing near to God by confession and repentance of sin. We draw near to Him when we are aware of our need for a Savior, when we pray in the name of Jesus who gives us access to the Father, when we read God's word and choose to believe those words. Faith comes to us by the hearing of God's word. Without such faith, it is impossible to please God. Additionally, we draw near to God by doing the words of God recorded in the Bible. This places us in a position before God's throne of grace to receive help and mercy.

The Spirit of God sees a sincere heart seeking after Him. He begins an inner work bringing confidence before Him, not based on our performance. God gives righteousness to us, based on the work of Jesus for our salvation. We are forgiven and freed from sin through faith and trust in Jesus Christ. His vicarious sacrifice pays the penalty for our sin.

The Spirit of God works this assurance of salvation in a way that only He can do in the heart and soul of one seeking Him. He confirms these truths in our hearts so that you know that you know that you have eternal life, that you are a child of God. The Holy Spirit is pleased to confirm in your spirit this assurance of your salvation.

We know this by revelation of the Holy Spirit as we have faith in Jesus and the Word of God. He will then also show evidence of His favor and forgiveness. He confirms this assurance of salvation through answers to prayer and experiences of His intervention. Signs, wonders, and answers to prayer will accompany those who believe, confirming saving faith in Jesus and assurance of eternal life. Signs and wonders also occur as a witness to the kingdom of God at hand for those who do not believe. Assurance of salvation is an essential requirement in participating in God's divine nature, escaping the corruption that is in the world, and growing in faith and authority as a believer.

The importance of this assurance of salvation is recorded in a story in the book of Acts. There were some people who were attempting to drive out demons in Jesus name. These seven sons of Sceva heard a reply from the demonic forces they were attempting to drive out, stating "I know Jesus and I Paul, but I do not know you." These were people attempting to do the works of God without the righteousness and power that comes from God to those who believe in Him and receive Him as their Lord and Savior. The demonic forces turned against them and left them bleeding and naked.[2]

In contrast to these seven sons of Sceva, Jesus sent out the 70 and told them to preach the word, heal the sick, cleanse lepers, and cast out demons. When they returned they rejoiced greatly and said that even the demons submit to them in Jesus name. Jesus replied, stating that they should rejoice that their names are written in the book of life.[3] The difference between the 7 sons of Sceva and the 70 followers of Jesus was that the 70 received Jesus, believed in Him and the good news of the gospel, had their names written in the book of life, and were sent out by Jesus and followed His instructions.

Receive the Power of the Holy Spirit

Acts 1:8 states, "But you shall receive power when the Holy Spirit has come upon you; and you shall be witnesses in Jerusalem and in all Judea and Samaria and to the end of the earth." Jesus made this promise of the Holy Spirit before the day of Pentecost. He instructed His disciples to wait before they go out because they needed to be clothed with power from on high. You would not go outside without clothes on; neither should a Christian go out to surrounding areas or to the ends of the earth without being clothed with power from on high.

When a person prays to invite Jesus into his heart, he gets a three-for-one deal. God, the Father, Jesus His Son, and the Holy Spirit enter. Holy Spirit enables an ability to say Jesus is Lord. After coming to saving faith in Jesus Christ, an additional encounter with the Holy Spirit brings the outpouring of His power.

The power of the Holy Spirit comes upon people in different ways and experiences. Some people grow up in the faith and do not have any particular dramatic experience of empowering, but are nonetheless truly filled with the power of the Holy Spirit. Most people report some kind of encounter with the empowering of the Holy Spirit, but these also can vary somewhat. Very often there are manifestations of this power such as speaking in tongues, prophesy, other gifts of the Holy Spirit, increased faith, desire for and understanding of God's word, deliverance and freedom from some areas of bondage, and inner spiritual power to live the Christian life. This power within the spirit filled believer accomplishes much. It is the same power that raised Jesus from the dead.

Our part is to yield to the Holy Spirit and not quench the Holy Spirit. We do this by setting our minds on the things of the Spirit and not on the things of the flesh. The Holy Spirit gives power to believers for witness to others, for building up the church, and for personal edification. This baptism of the Holy Spirit is to be received by every believer for the purposes of letting it out to benefit others and advance God's kingdom.

Abiding

1 John 2:21: "the anointing which you received from him abides in you." If you have been saved and filled with the Holy Spirit, you probably remember some times in the past when you were especially aware of this power being present within you and going out from you. Here is the good news of this Scripture: this same power remains within you no matter whether you feel it or not. The anointing that you noticed in the past remains with you; it abides in you. You may need to repent and to return to healthy spiritual disciplines and stir up the spiritual gifts within you. You may be continuing faithfully in your Christian walk, but are not feeling anything special at the moment. Nevertheless, His anointing abides in you. When you begin to minister to someone, you may be reminded of some obscure sin of yours or some shortcoming in the past. Remember you are forgiven and cleansed by Jesus' blood shed on the cross, and His anointing you received from Him abides in you.

Romans 11:29 states that the gift and calling of God are without repentance. This Scripture specifically references Paul's statements about God's chosen people, the people of Israel. God's call and election is now extended to all people and remains upon the ones that are called according to His purpose. God does not change His mind – His gifts and calling upon you remain.

Outpouring of Power

The disciples that Jesus had already sent forth in His name to perform great signs and wonders were the same disciples Jesus instructed to wait in Jerusalem until they were closed with power from on high. These disciples had seen God's power for healing and deliverance as they went out in Jesus' name. They saw great miracles occurring as they went out two by two. However, these disciples had not yet received the Holy Spirit's power. They went out in Jesus' name, but not yet empowered by the Holy Spirit. It was better for them not to go until they received power given by the Holy Spirit. This empowering and outpouring of the Holy Spirit was foundational for Jesus' disciples to go forth in His name. To live the Christian life and be effective witnesses nearby and far off requires the power of the Holy Spirit.

They did wait in Jerusalem and, on the day of Pentecost, they received the power of the Holy Spirit. Most of them, however, remained in Jerusalem and did not go out. Acts 1.8 says you shall receive power when the Holy Spirit has come upon you, and you shall be my witnesses in Jerusalem, Judea, Samaria, and to the ends of the earth. The Holy Spirit did come with power to those people on the day of Pentecost and numerous occasions thereafter (and down through the ages to this day). They did receive power but they remained in Jerusalem. They did not any time soon go out to become witnesses in Judea, Samaria, and to the ends of the earth. Acts 8:1 says that a great persecution arose so that the believers were scattered throughout the region. It was persecution that brought the believers to scatter and spread the gospel.

Acts 1:8 or 8:1? If you are wondering where is the anointing that you once received, experienced, or operated in, then return to going out as witnesses for Jesus Christ. Start doing the stuff of the gospel again. If you are not hearing God's guidance, go back to doing the Word of God; go back to what He last told you to do and be sure you obey those words. There are plenty of instructions in the Scriptures to occupy our time. Be doers of the word, not hearers only. Those who receive the power of the Holy Spirit should understand that this is not just for our own edification; this power is to be given out to others for salvation, healing, and deliverance.

Romans 8:11 says that the same power that raised Jesus from the dead dwells in us. This is worth repeating: the same power that raised Jesus from the dead dwells in us. This is something you should regularly call to mind and confess outwardly. Freely we have received this power and freely we are to give it to others. Let's understand this great power that dwells in believers and learn how to let it out to others for salvation, healing, and deliverance.

How can you receive this outpouring of the power of the Holy Spirit? Most commonly this occurs when another Spirit empowered believer prays for you with the laying on of hands. Some people pray alone and receive the Spirit's power, but the witness of scriptural accounts of the outpouring of power of the Holy Spirit occur through the ministry of believers, one to another.

How can you minister the baptism and empowering of the Holy Spirit to another person? How can you pray for yourself for this to occur in your life? First, I lead in a prayer of repentance and forgiveness. Unrepentance and unforgiveness will hinder the release of the Holy Spirit's power. This can be a simple statement of repentance and request for forgiveness. Secondly, I lead the person to renounce the devil and all his works and ways. Thirdly, I request the power of the Holy Spirit, the baptism of the Holy Spirit. Jesus said, "If even sinful persons like yourselves know how to give good gifts to your children, how much more will your Heavenly Father give the Holy Spirit to those who ask him" Luke 11:13. And lastly, I help them receive the power of the Holy Spirit by giving thanks. There are four components to this prayer ministry: Repent; Renounce; Request; Receive. Then I often pray in the Spirit with my hands placed upon the person's head or shoulder. Here, then, is how you might lead another person in prayer, having them repeat your words as you guide the prayer for the outpouring of the Holy Spirit's power:

> Father in heaven, I repent of my sins and commit my life to you and your will. I ask you to forgive me of all my sins. I forgive anyone who has sinned against me. I renounce and reject the devil. In the name of Jesus, I break any power assignments or strongholds that are not of God. Now I ask for the baptism of the Holy Spirit and fire. I ask for the empowering of the Holy Spirit along with the fruits and gifts of the Holy Spirit. I ask for this in Jesus name, laying claim to your promise to pour out your Spirit on all flesh. I thank you for the power of the Holy Spirit. I receive this gift of the Holy Spirit with thanksgiving. I pray this in the name of Jesus Christ. Amen.

Chapter 3

Let the Power Out

The Scriptures report that those who believe in Jesus have within them the same power that raised Jesus from the dead. Romans 8:11 states: "If the Spirit of him who raised Jesus from the dead dwells in you, He who raised Christ Jesus from the dead will give life to your mortal bodies also through His Spirit which dwells in you."

Power Within

Are you aware of this great truth? Do you realize and understand that those who believe in Jesus and are filled with the Holy Spirit have resurrection power within? That's a lot of power. Most believers do not know this or believe it. The challenge for the church is to know this resurrection power within and learn how to let it out to further God's kingdom. The Scriptures speak very clearly about this, but most believers do not know about and use the tools we are given. Let's strive to understand how to let this resurrection power go forth to accomplish not our own desires, but God's will.

> "...that I might know Him and the power of his resurrection, and may share in his suffering becoming like Him in his death, that if possible I may attain the resurrection from the dead. Not that I have already obtained this or am already perfect, but I press on to

make it my own, because Christ Jesus has made me his own" Philippians 3:10-12.

There are forty-one stories in the synoptic Gospels[1] about Jesus and His disciples ministering healing to the sick. If you look closely at each one of these episodes, not once did Jesus or His disciples pray. There was one time where the disciples had difficulty driving the demon out of a young boy, when Jesus stated this kind only comes out by prayer and fasting. However, Jesus did not pray or fast then when He drove out the demon. He was talking about the lifestyle of abiding in the Father. James 5:14-16 provides another reference to prayer and healing. Those who are sick are to call upon the elders of the church and let them pray the prayer of faith and the Lord will raise them up. This "prayer of faith" describes what we see Jesus and His disciples doing in those 41 stories of healing recorded in the Gospels.

Release This Power

Certainly prayer works. There are many promises in the Scriptures regarding prayer. It's a wonder how little we pray when we have such great promises, but this was not the method that Jesus or His disciples used when letting the power out to bring healing to other people. Prayer and fasting is essential to abiding in the Father and being filled and empowered with the Holy Spirit, but when the time came to let that power out, Jesus and His disciples did not pray.

When the disciples asked the Lord to increase their faith, Jesus answered speaking about faith as a grain of mustard seed and saying to this mountain, 'move from here to there', and it will be done. Jesus instructed them and us to speak to these objects that have no ears and cannot hear. We do not regularly speak this way. We are not accustomed to speaking to inanimate objects or things that we cannot converse with, but this is exactly what Jesus told us to do.

Instead the church prays, "Lord you move the mountain, you move the mulberry tree, you move the sycamine tree". Then Jesus says, "No, I said that you can speak to these and they will obey you." Then the church says, "All power and glory beyond belong to you, please move the mountain." Jesus again says, "No, I said you can move the mountain. I have given you authority to move the mountain." The church says, "No, you move it, we cannot move a mountain." And so the people of God keep asking God to do what He told them to do. Jesus said we, with the faith of a mustard seed, will ourselves speak to the mountain commanding it to move. Jesus tells us how to release His resurrection power within us when He says that we will say to the mountain, move from here to there and it will move.

Some people might speak to their plants. Certainly we have talked to our pets. A dog can understand us to a certain degree because they have ears to hear and they have eyes to watch and perceive. However, we are not accustomed to speaking to inanimate things without ears or an ability to understand. If you have tried something like this, at first it feels strange. If you look closely at Scripture and understand the power and authority given to believers, it is what Jesus taught and demonstrated.

God created the heavens and the earth by His word, speaking commands to create what exists out of nothing. We, who are created in the image of God, when redeemed by Jesus' shed blood and filled with the Holy Spirit, are authorized to do the same type of thing. We are functioning as God's children, created in His image, when we so speak.

Stop Praying

Have you ever tried to stop praying when you minister healing to someone? We are so accustomed to praying for healing. This will take a conscious effort to stop praying to God and start speaking to the disease or infirmity.

God spoke to Moses as recorded in Exodus 14:15: "Why do you cry to me? Tell the people of Israel to go forward." God told the Hebrew people to stop praying, start marching, and not fear the Egyptians who were pursuing them. God could have Himself held the waters back for the people to cross the Red Sea. Instead He had Moses lift up his rod and stretch out his hand over the waters for God's power to be released for their deliverance from Pharaoh and the Egyptians.

There is a time to pray, but when it is time to release the power within us who believe, prayer, though it can be effective, is not the method that Jesus taught. If you know you are going to say to a blind person, "Receive your sight," it makes you want to pray to prepare yourself and be filled with the Holy Spirit. So prayer is a foundation for ministering healing to other people, but when it was time to release the power that raised Jesus from the dead that dwells in believers, prayer was not the method that Jesus taught and demonstrated. His disciples then imitated Jesus methods when they ministered healing. There is no recorded Scripture of Jesus' disciples praying for the sick. There are a few instances in Scripture when the disciples did pray just before ministering healing. (See Acts 9:40 and 28:8.)

This extends beyond the ministry of healing. Jesus' instructions about faith involved speaking to a mountain or sycamine tree. These instructions are relevant to any area of authority given to believers. (This is unpacked in the 2nd section of this book).

I was discussing these matters with the person outside of a building that our church owned at the state fair. This is a building where a cup of water was given to those who wish to receive, providing an opportunity for ministry and evangelism. At the time that this building was scheduled to close, a few of us were talking about the authority that believers have. One of the volunteers inside stated that there was a bat inside and she needed help to get it out before we could close the building. Then one of them said to me, "Well, there is your opportunity to demonstrate how this works." So often we like to talk about these matters without doing them. Honestly, I was more interested in talking about it than demonstrating the authority we have. As I was summoned to demonstrate, I walked into the building and spoke to that bat, commanding it to leave the building in Jesus name. Immediately the bat flew in front of us and directly out the door.

There are numerous ways in the Scriptures by which Jesus and His disciples let the power of God out. Most commonly it was through word of command and laying on of hands. Sometimes it was simply faith in action. Occasionally there are reports of more extraordinary means such as handkerchiefs, aprons, mud, and even the shadow of

Peter passing over the people as he walked near them. Start by using these methods of laying on of hands and word of command in very simple ways. You can speak to your own body where you may need healing. Start with something simple like a headache. Speak to the headache pain and command it to leave in Jesus name.

The Scriptures teach this strategy for letting out that resurrection power within believers. The Word of God records seven times where Jesus told us that we would speak to the mountain (or the mulberry tree or the sycamine tree) and it would obey us. These statements came after a request by the apostles for increased faith. Jesus said this kind of faith is small like a mustard seed. It is not mustered up faith; it is mustard seed faith. We release God's resurrection power by speaking to a specific matter, giving a word of command in the name of Jesus. The most common method used to minister healing to others occurs through the laying on of hands and word of command.

Of course, prayer brings results. It's good to pray. We should pray fervently and often. Then we can use our authority as believers. We are created in the image of God with the ability to speak words with the authority given to us. From the beginning, God spoke to create the heavens and the earth. In a much smaller way, but essential for blessings others and advancing God's Kingdom, we are to speak with authority to bring salvation, deliverance, and healing to others. We are functioning then within the realm of what we were created to be and do.

Upon learning these truths, I made a distinct, conscious decision to try to stop praying when ministering healing to others. It forced me to do what Jesus told us to do. It did not seem natural. I was speaking to things that do not communicate, that do not have ears to hear me. Jesus taught His disciples to do this in order to release this great power within. When I began to speak to "this mountain," I soon began to see a notable increase in results.

Chapter 4

Replace the Light Bulb

———————————◦———————————

E veryone believes in electricity. It's not often that we actually see electricity, but we usually see what it can do. No one questions the existence of electricity. We believe in electricity because we frequently see what it does. Electrical current powers almost everything that we regularly use that requires energy. For a relatively short time in the span of history, we have enjoyed the benefits of electricity when controlled and employed to power various appliances and tools. Before the time of Thomas Edison and Benjamin Franklin, electricity was seen as lightning and static electricity, as we can still observe occasionally today.

An Electrical Circuit

Though we do not usually see electricity directly, everyone has come to believe that it exists and has power to accomplish various things. So when a light switch is turned on, we expect light to fill the room. When light does not occur despite throwing the switch, no one would think of imploring electricity to work, saying "O Electricity, I believe in you. I've seen you work in the past and do mighty things. Please come again now so this light will work."

Instead, when the light does not come on, we might first think that the light bulb has burned out. If we replace the light bulb and the light still does not come on, no one would stop and speak to electricity, calling upon it to work once again. Rather, we might think the circuit breaker has been tripped, the switch is faulty, or the wiring has a short.

If somehow we as a society decided that electricity was no longer needed or we neglected to teach our children about its benefits and how it works, after a few centuries it could be that people would have difficulty believing electricity could do all the things that we currently experience.

How absurd this discussion about electricity seems to us. This parallels how most Christians think about healing and miracles. The Scriptures say that heaven and earth will pass away, but God's word will not pass away. These same Scriptures teach that God through Jesus Christ is Savior and Healer. What we encounter with our natural senses will pass away. The forever Word of God as written in the Bible is truer than the natural world in which we live. Jesus said that people are ever seeing, but not perceiving; ever hearing, but not understanding. The wonders and intricacies of creation, speak loudly to a loving, able creator, yet we question His willingness to heal despite the marvels of creation and the truths of Scripture.

A Spiritual Circuit

Almost 20% of the verses in the four gospels of Matthew, Mark, Luke, and John have to do with testimonies of and discussion about healing. We see in these and other Scriptures that healing is in the atonement, that is to say, that Jesus' death and resurrection purchased healing for our bodies. Surely He has borne our sicknesses and taken our diseases. By His stripes we are healed.[1]

These Scriptures about how to minister healing have not been taught adequately. Over many centuries the neglect of teaching these truths has caused us to question and doubt God's will to heal. All along the need for healing continues everywhere. Virtually everyone has been ill and needed healing at some time or another during a lifespan. Most Christians believe God can heal. We pray and implore God to heal, but healings occur infrequently or not at all for most people. Many conclude that God can heal, but does not heal very often nowadays.

Various doctrines have arisen to explain this. Some have concluded that signs and wonders no longer occur because they were done only to establish the early church. Some even state that God sends diseases and illnesses to people to teach them a lesson. We would never think of sending our children to a school where the teachers inflicted illness on the students so that they could learn some lessons. Yet people describe God in this way.

God does work all things together for good with those who love Him and are called according to His purpose. He does work through human sufferings and sicknesses to bring about His greater purpose because He is the great Redeemer. I injured my knee, a torn MCL ligament, when playing intramural football. When I learned that I would be in a cast and using crutches for six weeks, I asked God what good he would work in these circumstances. The thought occurred to me immediately: "Now that you cannot walk (physically), I will teach you to walk (spiritually)." Throughout those six weeks I was reminded of my spiritual walk with every time I employed my crutches to walk physically. God was redeeming these circumstances and working them for his good purposes.

We read about the God of wonders in the Scriptures, but most do not experience Him this way today. We believe God has power to heal but we struggle with unbelief because we simply do not see enough evidence of supernatural healing. It may seem God's healing light does not turn on when we try to turn on the switch. So we question God's will to heal. Instead, we should question how healing works and learn from the eternal Word of God how God's people release His power.

Jesus showed frustration with His disciples, stating that He had been with them long enough, when they were not able to bring healing to the boy who was demonized.[2] There was no question in this discussion about God's power or willingness to heal. Jesus challenged His disciples to follow Him and learn how to release the power of God within believers.

When the light bulb does not turn on, we do not question electricity. When healing does not happen, we should not question God's will or power. Rather we should consider how healing works and where the interruption of God's flow of power may occur. When a fluorescent light does not work it may be a problem with the ballast. It's unnecessary to replace the whole circuitry providing power to the lightbulb to fix the problem. An electrician can restore light by attending to a specific problem such as the ballast. If the ballast is replaced and the light still does not come on, the electrician does not give up and conclude that electricity is no longer real or willing to light the bulb. He will look next at the switch, the wiring, or the light bulb. None of us would conclude, when a light does not work, that electricity is not real or able to provide light. Rather we look for a problem in the flow of electricity.

Neither should we doubt God's power and willingness to heal. Rather we should look at the conduit through which God's healing flows. Healing occurs when we release the power of God dwelling in us through the laying on of hands and word of command. The power inside of a Spirit-filled Christian is the same power that raised Jesus from the dead. We let this power out through the laying on of hands and words of command, to speak to and move "this mountain."

God Heals Through His People

God rarely heals sovereignly. He has restricted His healing power to flow through believers who are filled with the Holy Spirit and know how to minister healing. Instructions in James regarding sickness clarify God's intended flow of healing power.

> "Is any among you sick? Let them call upon the elders of the church, and let them pray over him, anointing him with oil in the name of the Lord; and the prayer of faith will save the sick man, and the Lord will raise him up; and if he is committed sins, he will be forgiven. Therefore confess your sins to one another, and pray for one another, that you may be healed" James 5:14-16.

If God did heal sovereignly without sending His transcendent power through certain vessels, then there was no need for Jesus to send out the seventy and instruct them to preach and heal. Healings occurred when they did go and preach the good news. If for some reason they did not go, those healings would not have happened. God does not often heal apart from working through the body of believers.

Jesus understood God's plan to minister through His people. This was the primary reason why Jesus chose twelve disciples and why He sent out the seventy. He instructed these disciples in the things of the kingdom of God. Jesus was frustrated with His disciples when they could not yet bring healing to the demonized boy. He was disturbed about this knowing that the extension of God's compassion for His people would come through His people. If the disciples of Jesus could not bring healing to others, God would not bypass them to heal anyway. Healing occurs through the body of believers.

Jesus said it is better for Him to go to the Father, because the Father would send the Holy Spirit to increase the same works that He did, now through Spirit-filled believers. This clearly demonstrates God's intent that, through the church, these blessings would go forth. If the church is not releasing these blessings from God, it is not because God has changed from His generous and merciful plans.

Because most Christians do not understand how to let the power out and minister healing, many have come to question whether God wishes to heal. Doctrines of sickness and illness then arise attempting to explain this, saying that God has some larger purpose for sickness and illness that they must accept.

The Scriptures are abundantly clear regarding God's provision for healing. This provision is still available for us today. When believers, filled with the Holy Spirit, release the resurrection power within them to those in need, then God's provision for healing is engaged. So we must learn from the Scriptures what faith is and how to release the power that Jesus places in us. We must learn to speak to "this mountain" and see it move for God's purposes and for His glory. When the healing light of God does not shine, we should consider where, in the circuitry of God's electrical healing power, might this healing power be interrupted.

Chapter 5

We Give You What We Have

A man unable to walk from his birth was being carried to the entrance of the gate called Beautiful. As Peter and John walked by, he began to ask for money as this was apparently his only means of acquiring income. Peter and John gave him some attention by looking at him and the man expected to receive some money. Then Peter and John said something to him that is instructive for us.

> "Now Peter and John were going up to the temple at the hour of prayer, the ninth hour. And a man lame from birth was being carried, whom they laid daily at that gate of the temple which is called Beautiful to ask alms of those who entered the temple. Seeing Peter and John about to go into the temple, he asked for alms. And Peter directed his gaze at him, with John, and said, "Look at us." And he fixed his attention upon them, expecting to receive something from them. But Peter said, "I have no silver and gold, but I give you what I have; in the name of Jesus Christ of Nazareth, walk." And he took him by the right hand and raised him up; and immediately his feet and ankles were made strong. And leaping up he stood and walked and entered the temple with them, walking and leaping and praising God" Acts 3:1-8.

I Give You What I Have

"I have no silver and gold, but I give you what I have; in the name of Jesus Christ of Nazareth, walk." Peter said he did not have silver and gold but he was going to give something that he did have. Peter and John were aware of something that they had and they knew how to give it to him. Most Christians are not aware of what they have and do not know how to give it to someone else. We do know how to give money, but we do not know how to give what Peter and John gave. Most Christians do not know that they have something they can give besides money and material things. This lame man's healing would likely remedy his needs for money or material things. Peter and John gave healing to him.

What did Peter and John have? They knew that they had the power of the Holy Spirit within them and they knew that they could give healing to this man. They knew that God had given it to them to give to him. Healing comes from God and He has given it to believers to give to others. It was now theirs to give to this paralytic man.

Many people do not understand this truth. They do not recognize that Christians have something given to them by God. Instead some might ask God to give healing to someone. Some may think in today's world only the doctors and medically trained people can assist the body in its own built in healing abilities. Others ask for God's grace and strength to endure, without any request for healing. Missing is an awareness of the great truth that the same power that raised Jesus from the dead dwells in believers.

Note that Peter did not say that God would give healing to him. He said, "I give you what I have." Through the Holy Spirit, God empowers the hands and words of believers. Now the church has the opportunity, the call, and the duty to give to those in need. Peter and John are saying that God has given healing to believers. All believers are to freely give what they have freely received. Peter and John were obeying what Jesus told them to do: "Heal the sick, raise the dead, cleanse lepers, cast out demons. You received without paying, give without pay." Matthew 10:8.

How To Give What You Have

Furthermore, Peter and John knew how to give this gift to this lame man. They did it by word of command and they took him by the arm and raised him up. So it involved words and touch. When we speak in the name of Jesus, based on the authority given to us to heal, power goes forth. When we lay hands on people in the name of Jesus, we release what has been given to us and give it to another person. Power goes forth in the laying on of hands in the name of Jesus. Peter touched him by taking his hand. He also used this connection to assist the man in raising him up. Through this process and means, God's healing power was given to this paralytic.

This lame man came every day to this gate looking for money, but he was healed ONLY on the day that these two Spirit-filled Christians encountered him. These two knew what they had to give and how to give it to him. For all the other days that he came to this gate when no miracle happened, it would have been easy to erroneously conclude that God does not want to heal or no longer heals. One could conclude that there was some sin he or his parents committed. Others could determine God should not heal because it would show favoritism to this man when there are others who are not healed. Why was he healed on this particular day and not the day before or two days before or any other day of his life? Did God not want to heal him except for that particular day? He was healed on that day because two believers, who knew what they had and how to give it, brought God's healing to him. There was nothing special about that day versus any other day. Any day when Peter and John would pass by him and give them what they had would suffice.

On the day when Jesus sent out the seventy to preach the good news and heal the sick, they did go out and did bring healing to those needing it. Even the demons fled in Jesus' name. Had those seventy not gone on that day, there would not have been report of many spontaneous healings in the path they were to walk on. Had they gone the next day instead, the report would have been the same. Those healings occurred because those seventy commissioned by Jesus went out and gave what they had.

Go With Nothing and Freely Give

Jesus told them to freely give as they had freely received. When He told them to go, He instructed them to take no money or extra clothes or material things.[1] What did they have to give if they took nothing with them? Jesus told them to give freely, but they were to take nothing with them. He told them to go, preach, teach, and heal the sick. Had they brought material things with them, the focus could easily shift to these possessions and away from their commission. The disciples and those receiving ministry from them can be distracted away from God's provision and commands. Peter said to the paralytic, "Look at us." This man was accustomed to hope for alms from anyone who would give him some attention. In saying, "Look at us", Peter was calling him away from this focus and wanted him to hear his words and receive what he had to give.

Healing happens when believers understand what they have and know how to give it to others. It's the same message given to Abraham: "I will make of you a great nation, and I will bless you, so that you will be a blessing" Genesis 12:2. Jesus said it's better for Him to go to the Father because the Holy Spirit will be given to believers to exponentially multiply His ministry. God wants to see people healed and has given this ministry to the church.

One of God's names in the Old Testament is Jehovah Raphah, meaning "The Lord your healer". His nature is to heal and restore; healing is woven into his Name. His heart aches for His church to understand, believe, and give out the same ministry Jesus brought.

Unlike the vast majority of Christians today, Peter and John knew they had something to give this paralytic. It was not silver or gold; it was not material things. Not only did they have something to give him, they knew how to give it to him. God healed this man because a couple of Spirit-filled believers brought healing to him in the name of Jesus and to the glory of God.

How many Christians today would be able to say what Peter and John said? You might rather hear different words such as: "I can't help you with your paralysis, but here's some money;" or "Here's some money, would you mind if I prayed for you to ask God if He would bless you?" There's no harm in this; it does bring blessings to others, but it typifies a common lack of knowledge of what great power God has given to believers and how this power is given for healing, deliverance, and salvation. Most do not realize they have healing to give to others. Most also do not know how to give it to those needing healing.

These instructions Jesus gave to His disciples are the same for believers today. In the Great Commission of Matthew 28, He told those disciples to go and make disciples of all nations and teach them to do what Jesus taught them to do. Jesus taught His disciples to go, preach, teach, and heal. Specifically, Christians today then are to go, preach, teach, and heal just as His disciples were taught by Him and were told to disciple others to do.

Chapter 6

Laws Guide Us or Break Us

M y college roommate recounted how as a child he learned obedience from his parents. He tried several times to cross boundaries set by his parents. He was told not to go past a certain landmark near his home, but he was permitted to play in his yard in the area that his parents established. He stated that it seemed every time he crossed over the boundary, his parents somehow found out about it and they gently and firmly called him to account for his behavior. Looking back on this, he saw God at work through his parents. He concluded that God made a way for his parents to know when he crossed the boundaries, thereby teaching him obedience through his parents.

As part of my pastoral education, I was assigned to a hospital setting. On occasion I was called as a chaplain to the Emergency Department when a significant tragedy or trauma occurred. Over the two months of time spent there, I noted that every tragedy to which I was called had some connection with breaking the law. One young man was driving drunk and hit a tree, leaving him paralyzed from below his waist. Another man was hunting deer out of season and just past sundown. His hunting partner thought he saw a deer and shot his friend through the neck leaving him with quadriplegia.

Not every misbehavior or law-breaking results in calamity or tragedy. There are plenty of life's events that have no apparent connection to wrongdoing. "Many are the afflictions of the righteous, but the Lord delivers him out of them all" Psalm 34:19. Jesus suffered despite being without sin, learning obedience through His sufferings.[1] The real test is not whether we suffer, but did we learn obedience through our sufferings. Where laws are broken, there may be consequences, as most laws exist for our protection. We really do not break laws, they break us. The consequences for violating laws come back upon the ones guilty of them.

Types of Laws

There are different types of laws: spiritual laws; physical laws; societal laws; and relationship laws. Various laws are interconnected and at times involve more than one category.

There are spiritual laws that transcend all cultures and all time. They are established by God and based on His truth. Spiritual laws are more intangible, relating to the spirit and soul and not always directly or immediately related to physical nature or matter. Examples include the Ten Commandments, love one another, death as the penalty for sin, and the law of spirit and life in Christ Jesus, which has set us free from the law of sin and death.

There are also thousands of laws that govern our behavior in society. These societal laws include criminal laws, civil laws, common laws, and statuate laws. Some examples here include speed limits, laws related to financial transactions and investments, and fishing and hunting limits.

And there are physical laws. These are laws that God has built into His creation. They are amazingly connected and interactive. Examples are the law of gravity, thermodynamics, and fluid dynamics among many others.

Consider the physical law of gravity, a force that God has created between two objects. Every mass has an inherent quality of attraction called gravity. The mass of our earth is so large that it holds everything on its surface (unless enough force is applied to overcome the force of the Earth's gravity). As children we learn to function within the law of gravity. We learn to obey the law of gravity. Learning to walk, run, and ride a bicycle involves many falls because of gravity. Suppose a person concluded that he did not like gravity, or did not believe in gravity, or concluded that, though it may work for other people, it does not work for him. If this person decided to jump from the roof of his house, we all know that he would fall despite his beliefs, feelings, rationalizations, and conclusions.

The Hebrew usage of the word 'law' is almost synonymous with 'teaching.' The Bible speaks of great blessings for those who learn and obey the law, the teaching of the Lord. And the Scriptures warn those who disregard these laws. "If one turns away his ear from hearing the law, even his prayer is an abomination" Proverbs 28:9.

These laws are not intended to restrict but to protect. All of us have violated laws; we are all guilty of sin. There are associated consequences in this life and for eternity. The good news of the gospel is that Jesus paid the price for our sins. The law of forgiveness overcomes the law of condemnation for those who are in Christ Jesus. "There is therefore now no condemnation for those who are in Christ Jesus. For the law of the spirit and life in Christ Jesus has set me free from the law sin and death" Romans 8:1-2.

Laws of Ministry

There are laws and instructions regarding ministering healing and releasing the resurrection power that dwells within believers. These laws and instructions supersede and overcome the natural process of sin and sickness. Learning these principles and obeying these instructions invoke and enable a higher "law" of righteousness, peace, and joy in the Holy Spirit.

An airplane in flight seems to defy gravity. As you know, the force of gravity is still functioning as usual. Other physical laws of aerodynamics overcome the force of gravity allowing an airplane to fly. Similarly, a Spirit-filled believer can learn the laws of Scripture and operate within these spiritual laws to overcome sickness and disease by God's power. So there are also "laws" or teachings regarding how faith and ministry occur.

There are certain laws that we can learn from the Scriptures regarding many aspects of life, including effective, powerful prayer and how forgiveness and healing work. When Spirit-filled believers are careful to understand the will of God and His instructions for ministering to others, greater works than Jesus did will occur, because He went to the Father and sent the Holy Spirit to teach us and empower us.

We must all learn obedience. Just as we benefit by learning to operate within the law of gravity, we benefit by learning obedience to God's laws in His word. We must be careful to obey the laws of God, the Word of God, and the specific leading of the Holy Spirit. There are many Scriptures that speak of obedience. Here are a few:

> "Be very careful, then, how you live – not as unwise but as wise, making the most of every opportunity, because the days are evil. Therefore do not be foolish, but understand what the Lord's will is" Ephesians 5:15-17.

> "He who has my commandments and keeps them, he it is who loves me; and he who loves me will be loved by my Father, and I will love him and show myself to him" John 14:21.

> "As obedient children, do not be conformed to the passions of your former ignorance, but as he who called you is holy, be holy yourselves in all your conduct" 1 Peter 1:14.

> "Having purified your souls by your obedience to the truth for a sincere love of the brethren, love one another earnestly from the heart" 1 Peter 1:22.

> "Through whom we have received grace and apostleship to bring about the obedience of faith for the sake of his name among all the nations" Romans 1:5.

> "Do you not know that if you yield yourselves to any one as obedient slaves, you are slaves of the one whom you obey, either of sin, which leads to

death, or of obedience, which leads to righteousness?"
Romans 6:16.

"He who believes in the Son has eternal life; he who
does not obey the Son shall not see life, but the wrath
of God rests upon him" John 3:36.

"And we are witnesses to these things, and so is the
Holy Spirit whom God has given to those who obey
him" Acts 5:32.

These are just some of the many verses depicting the centrality
of obedience to God and His word. The Greek word for faith, pistis
(pistis), means equally faith and obedience. When we are careful to
obey God and His Word, we are expressing faith and love to Him.

Hear and Obey

We can best position ourselves to hear God first by looking to His
word written in the Scriptures, then by deciding, even before we hear
what He says, that we will obey. Our hearing is sharpened by such
trusting obedience of our heavenly Father. This submission to our
heavenly Father's plan is the safest and most fulfilling way to live.
Such obedience causes an increase of faith; such obedience is faith.
"My sheep hear my voice and they follow me" (John 10:10). If
you are not hearing God's voice, you should question if you are one
of His sheep. We can always hear God when we read the Bible, but
without the Spirit of Jesus opening our minds to the Word, the truths
of the Scriptures are hidden from unbelievers so that though hearing,
they are never perceiving or understanding.

"But, as it is written, "What no eye has seen, nor ear
heard, nor the heart of man conceived, what God has
prepared for those who love him," God has revealed
to us through the Spirit...Now we have received not
the spirit of the world, but the Spirit which is from

God, that we might understand the gifts bestowed on
us by God" 1 Corinthians 2:9-10, 12.

This is how we find truth: by obeying and doing God's word.
Anyone can find that Jesus' teaching is true by doing God's will.
Nothing is stated here about taking classes, understanding it first, or
feeling right about it first. Simply be a doer of the word and not a
hearer only. "Anyone who chooses to do the will of God will find
out whether my teaching comes from God or whether I speak on my
own" John 7:17.

When the apostle's asked the Lord for increased faith, Jesus
answer was simply a discussion about obedience. A disciple of Jesus
acquires increased faith by doing his duty. The book of James states:
faith is completed by works, by obedience to the Word of God.

> "What does it profit, my brethren, if a man says he has
> faith but has not works? Can his faith save him? If a
> brother or sister is ill-clad and in lack of daily food,
> and one of you says to them, "Go in peace, be warmed
> and filled," without giving them the things needed for
> the body, what does it profit? So faith by itself, if it
> has no works, is dead" James 2:14-17.

Abraham's faith expressed itself in willingness to offer his Son,
Isaac, the promise of God, upon an altar. His obedience brought him
to act upon God's command to sacrifice his only son that he loved,
despite certain confusion and questions why God would command
him to sacrifice the fulfillment of what He had previously promised
Abraham: through his offspring God would make a great nation that
would bless the world.

Moses obeyed everything the Lord commanded him. The phrase
"...as the Lord had commandment Moses" occurs about 80 times
in the Bible. Moses was careful to obey everything the Lord commanded him. Moses' obedience to the Lord was his one attribute that
enabled him to lead God's chosen people, see the Lord work mighty
miracles, and even see the back side of God.

Hebrews 11 is the great chapter of faith. It describes the actions of faith of many people as recorded in the Scriptures. All the people and events of faith listed involve action. Faith is not simply a set of beliefs. Faith moves us to act and obey. Faith in God is obedience to His Word. Faith is obedience to the law of the Lord, the teaching of the Lord. Understanding and obeying the laws and teachings recorded in the Scripture bring great blessings to many.

Chapter 7

Increase Our Faith

Faith is a big word with many facets and definitions. It is used in many ways and is directed toward many different objects and people. You might even know someone whose name is 'Faith'. Faith is not so easily defined because of its many uses and references. One can have faith in oneself, faith in another person, faith in God, faith that a chair will hold you up if you sit on it, faith that a bridge will not collapse if you drive over it. We might have faith in a sports team or a politician.

We use the word 'faithfulness' to refer to reliability and dependability. We also speak about 'keeping the faith,' which can refer to a set of agreed upon beliefs that are adhered to with perseverance. We talk about 'walking by faith' by plotting a course that has some unknown outcomes or following certain principles. Faith does involve an element of trust where one must depend on someone or something else. The early theologians said faith involves trust, intellectual assent, and commitment.

The Scriptures underscore the importance of faith. From the beginnings of Scripture, faith is established as the foundation of our relationship with the Father. "Abraham believed God and it was credited to him as righteousness, and he was called the friend of God" James 2:23. "The just shall live by faith" Habakkuk 2:4. Faith is the human response that establishes our righteousness before God. "Without faith it is impossible to please him. For whoever would draw near to God must believe that He exists and that He rewards those who seek him" Hebrews 11:6.

The Bible instructs us further about faith:

- Faith is the victory that overcomes the world.[1]
- Faith is more precious than gold.
- Through faith our eternal inheritance is guarded by God's power.
- Our faith is perishable and is tested by fire.
- The outcome of our faith brings us the salvation of our souls.[2]
- Faith is the assurance of things hoped for, the conviction of things not seen.[3]

Faith comes by hearing the word, focusing on the word, accepting the truth of the Word of God more than what you see with your eyes. What is yet unseen has more substance than what is seen with human eyes.

Believing is Seeing

There is an advertising slogan that says, "seeing is believing." The television ad depicts a product with desirable features, and then the observer is told to believe because of what was just seen. This is a truth that can be seen in Scripture. Jesus demonstrated the Kingdom of God by signs and wonders that the people saw and experienced. Many believed in Jesus and followed Him because of what they saw. Seeing was believing.

Jesus stated there was blessing for those who do not see and yet believe.[4] So this faith is where believing is seeing. Hebrews 11:1 states "faith is the assurance of things hoped for, the conviction of things not seen." This kind of faith was operating in Paul when he was first converted. He was blind after his encounter with Jesus on the Damascus Road. God then said to Ananias, "he (Paul) is praying, and *he has seen* a man named Ananias come in and lay his hands on him so that he might regain his sight" Acts 9:11-1 (Italics mine). Paul was blind at the time he was praying, yet he saw Ananias coming to him. This was Paul's eyes of faith. Believing was seeing.

Moses sent twelve men, one from each tribe, to explore the land of Canaan, the promised land. This was the land the Lord had promised the people as He led them out of Egyptian captivity. They all returned with a report of how the land was beautiful, flowing with milk and honey. Ten of the twelve also reported how the cities were well fortified and very large, how the people were powerful and of great size. "We seemed like grasshoppers in our own eyes, and we looked the same to them" Numbers 13:33. They were focused on what they saw and had seemingly forgotten the Lord's promise and the miraculous deliverances through which He already brought them. These ten men then spread a bad report to the Israelites about the promised land. They were unbelieving and therefore looked at the outward appearance and disregarded God's word of promise.

Two of the twelve, Joshua and Caleb, looking at the same people and land, returned with a different report. They stated to Moses and the people that they should go up and take possession of the land, for they could certainly do it. These two focused on the promise of God and awareness of His greatness. These two believers saw the same circumstances differently because of their faith. Their eyes of faith, based on the promise of God, enabled them to see differently than the other ten spies who looked at the giants. These two looked more at God's promise than what was seen in the natural. Believing was seeing.[5]

What is Faith?

Faith is based on the witness of the Scriptures describing what has been accomplished and given. 2 Peter 1:3 states "His divine power *has granted* to us all things that pertain to life and godliness" (Italics mine). So faith is looking back to lay claim to and appropriate what has already been given. Hope, however, is different from faith, as hope looks to the future, for something one does not yet have. "Now hope that is seen is not hope. For who hopes for what he sees? But if we hope for what we do not see, we wait for it with patience" Romans 8:24-25.

What is faith? Many have trouble defining faith. When people are asked, 'what is faith?,' some say 'faith is to believe in something.' When asked 'what is it to believe in something?,' some will say, 'to believe is to have faith.' So it is sometimes defined by a circular argument using synonyms without much depth or clarity. Because of its expanded meanings and uses, it is difficult to define faith. The importance of faith underscored in Scripture demands our study and attention, as the human response of faith is required for matters pertaining to this life and for eternity.

How do we grow in faith? How can a believer's faith be increased? Many think attending a bible study or a small fellowship group will increase faith. Maybe reading an inspirational book will increase faith. If you are hearing the Word of God in these activities, you can grow in faith. Faith comes by hearing, and hearing by the Word of God. We should not neglect to meet together for encouragement in the faith. However, Jesus never had His disciples enroll in a Bible study or classroom with homework. When He demonstrated and taught faith, He did not primarily engage the minds of His disciples to establish a cohesive systematic theology. We have often applied the didactic methods of our culture with the hope that faith will be increased.

Faith is Active

John 7 records how Jesus instructed the Jews that anyone can know if His teaching was from God, or if He was speaking on His own authority. He tells them how to know if His teaching is from God. The people were marveling that He had learning, but had never studied. Jesus' answer however was not about study or education. His response to them did not engage their minds, emotions, traditions, or experiences. He spoke to the human will. He said, "If any man's will is to do his will, he shall know whether the teaching is from God or whether I am speaking on my own authority" John 17:7. If any man's will is to DO God's will, he shall know... So in the Kingdom of God, knowledge comes by obedience. If you put God's words into practice, you will find that they are true and thereby acquire knowledge and wisdom. This is true regardless of understanding, agreement, feelings, traditions, or past experiences. If one sets His will to do God's will, even if not understanding it, not agreeing with it, not feeling up to it, not accustomed to it, but nevertheless chooses to do God's will, he will find that those words of Jesus are true. Obedience to the Word produces evidence of the Word.

Jesus repeatedly said that if we have a small amount of faith, as small as a mustard seed, we would be able to move mountains. So what is this faith? What can we learn from Jesus' explanations of faith? We do not see this kind of faith operating much among believers in the church. We do not see actual 'mulberry trees going into the sea' or 'mountains moving from here to there'. We do not often see figurative 'mulberry trees' or 'mountains' moving. What does Jesus teach His disciples about faith? The disciples who followed Jesus saw this great power of faith and how essential it was for life and for advancing God's kingdom. So they asked the Lord, 'increase our faith.' Jesus gave this answer in Luke 17:5-10:

> "The apostles said to the Lord, 'increase our faith!' And the Lord said, 'If you have faith as a grain of mustard seed, you could say to this sycamine tree, "Be rooted up, and be planted in the sea," and it would obey you. Will any one of you, who has a servant plowing or keeping sheep, say to him when he has come in from the field, "Come at once and sit down at table"? Will he not rather say to him, "Prepare supper for me, and gird yourself and serve me, till I eat and drink; and afterward you shall eat and drink? Does he thank the servant because he did what was commanded? So you also, when you have done all that is commanded you, say, 'We are unworthy servants; we have only done what was our duty'"" Luke 17:5-10.

Jesus talks about faith as small as a grain of mustard seed. It's a small seed that, when planted, grows large. What is this 'mustard seed' faith? Sometimes we might see 'mustered up' faith rather than mustard seed faith. Jesus never seems to muster up faith. He did not have to hype things up or engage people's emotions. It was not mustered up faith; it was mustard seed faith. So how does Jesus answer the apostle's quest for increased faith?

Jesus' Definition of Faith

Jesus could have responded with any of the many theological facets of faith. He did not address any of the good and sound ways faith is often defined as discussed above. He did not talk about trust or ascribing to a certain set of doctrines. He also did not talk about doubt. He did not chastise His apostles for asking this question, He rebuke them for a lack of faith.

Jesus defines faith in a way that is different than most people use today. He replied to their request for increased faith by discussing matters that few would use today to define or foster increased faith. I have asked many groups of believers to define faith. They all give good answers, but none in my experience have ever answered with these words Jesus used to instruct His apostles.

"If you have faith as a grain of mustard seed, you could say to this sycamine tree, 'Be rooted up, and be planted in the sea,' and it would obey you." Jesus answers their question by stating what the believer can say and do by virtue of their authority given to them and the power of their faith. We see this recorded seven times in the New Testament. With a small amount of faith we could say to a mountain, a sycamine tree, or a mulberry tree some word of command and it would obey US. He taught His apostle's about this faith that enables believers to speak a word of command to something to do something. The 'something' that is spoken to, will then obey.

God Speaks and We Speak

God displayed his nature and authority by speaking words to create the universe. Out of nothing, ex nihilo[6], all things were created by the spoken Word of God. The opening chapter of John's Gospel references Jesus as 'the Word of God.' The Son of God is the Word of God; the Word of God was spoken through Jesus with authority and power. Jesus was with God in the beginning and was involved in creation.

Humans were created by God, made in the image of God. What does it mean to be created in the image of God? We know it is God's nature, His image, His authority, to speak. What He said and says happens. We were created in that image. Human beings have the ability to speak language, unlike any other created species or thing. With mustard seed faith, a believer's words can also have supernatural power. He tells us to speak words in His name and with a small amount of faith. Thus we function as people created in the image of God.

Notice that Jesus told us to speak to inanimate things, things that do not have ears, cannot hear, and cannot understand what we are saying. The examples He uses are mountains and trees. No trees or mountains have interactive abilities to speak, reply, converse or understand. The nothingness that God spoke to before creation had no substance and thus no capability to respond. It was God's word that brought forth creation. The faith that Jesus teaches the apostles includes this kind of speech.

Faith is Obedience

One might think that Jesus finishes His answer to the apostle's quest for increased faith after making His statement about moving sycamine trees into the sea. The next verses continue His quoted answer. Jesus continues to answer their quest for increased faith as He talks about a servant working in the field and doing his duty. He spoke about this servant doing everything that was commanded him without any reciprocation or gratitude from the master. How does this relate to increased faith?

Jesus answers them by talking about two kinds of obedience. Jesus links faith with obedience. This obedience is directed in two different ways. He first talks about things that will obey us when we have faith. Secondly, He talks about being obedient to those in authority over us. He answers them by stating that faith is validated, empowered, and worked out first, by being obedient to those set over us, and secondly, by understanding and using our authority over things under our authority. Jesus answers their quest for faith by stating what we can say to a mountain and by doing our duty as a servant. Faith is closely connected to obedience, involving an understanding of and a functioning within the realms of the authority given to us. This teaching is essential for increased faith that moves mountains.

The Greek word for faith is 'pistis' (pistis). This word means equally faith and obedience. A simple, accurate, and profound definition of faith is this: faith is obedience. The apostle's asked about faith; Jesus answered with discussion about obedience.

The Centurion understood this truth. He stated to Jesus how he was under authority and in authority. Upon hearing him simply describing his position and authority, Jesus said that He had not found anyone in Israel with such great faith. It would have been more obvious for Jesus to say: never have I seen anyone in Israel with such great understanding of authority and obedience. Instead Jesus called it faith. The centurion spoke about obedience to authority and Jesus called this great faith.

> "As he entered Capernaum, a centurion came forward to him, beseeching him and saying, 'Lord, my servant is lying paralyzed at home, in terrible distress.' And he said to him, 'I will come and heal him.' But the centurion answered him, 'Lord, I am not worthy to have you come under my roof; but only say the word, and my servant will be healed. For I am a man under authority, with soldiers under me, and I say to one, "Go," and he goes, and to another, "Come," and he comes, and to my slave, "Do this, and he does it."' When Jesus heard him, he marveled, and said to those who followed him, "Truly, I say to you, not even in Israel have I found such faith" Matthew 8:5-10.

Jesus answered the apostle's quest for increased faith, stating the same things that He saw in the Centurion's faith. The Centurion understood authority. He understood the power of spoken words from those in authority. He knew Jesus had authority over his servant's paralysis. He knew Jesus could speak from His position of authority. He knew Jesus did not need to come near the paralyzed servant. It was not Jesus' position of proximity, but His position of authority to speak words of healing.

Jesus saw that the Centurion understood faith because he understood obedience and authority. The Centurion was under authority and careful to obey those set over him. He was thereby also in authority and could say to those in his battalion, "come, go, and do this or that," and they would obey him. The Centurion said he was a man under authority and he was able to say to those under his authority, 'go, do this, etc.' The Centurion spoke of obedience directed in two ways: obedience to those set over him, and obedience from those under his rule. This is exactly how Jesus answered the apostle's quest for increased faith. Jesus saw the Centurion understood obedience and authority so He complimented his great faith.

What is the authority that a believer in Jesus possesses? Just knowing this will bring increased faith. The Centurion knew these two facts: who he was under and who he was over. Your faith will increase by knowing your position in life, by knowing your place in the Kingdom of God. This is not an endeavor to somehow convince yourself that you believe God's Word without doubting. There is no requirement to become super spiritual or manufacture some elusive emotions or hype that might serve as faith. This is not a struggle to manipulate thoughts and feelings with the hope that somehow doubt will dissipate and faith will increase.

Faith is Authority

All of us are born into this world without much or any authority. As we grow and mature, we acquire certain positions of authority. The authority that you then acquire is instituted by God as all authority in earth is given by God. So what is this authority we acquire at home and work and what is the additional authority we acquire when believing in Jesus and submitting to Him as our Lord and Savior? Who are you subject to? Whose authority are you under? To know these is to increase your faith.

Most Christians do not really know the authority they have as believers. Of the few who do know their authority in Christ, most of them do not use it. We can know our position in this world and our position in the Kingdom of God. We can then function with confidence and with increased faith to use our authority for God's purposes. The Apostle Paul instructs us to think about ourselves with sober judgment according to the measure of faith (authority) God has assigned.

> "For by the grace given to me I bid every one among you not to think of himself more highly than he ought to think, but to think with sober judgment, each according to the measure of faith which God has assigned him" Romans 12:3.

Some indeed think too highly of themselves, taking pride in self rather than the commonwealth we have in heaven. Believers, who are crucified with Christ, therefore should deny themselves and think with sober judgment. Here then is where many think more lowly of themselves than they ought because they have not understood the measure of faith God has assigned them. They have not understood their position with Christ and the authority of the believer.

The "measure of faith which God has assigned him" is best understood in the context of Jesus' teaching about increased faith. The assigned measure of faith from God is the assigned position of authority given by God. God gives faith to believers; God gives authority to believers. We can know the measure of faith assigned us by knowing the position and authority given to us by God. We can find answers to this throughout Scripture. The following chapters explore just this. Your faith will increase by knowing what the Bible states about your position and authority as a believer. When you understand the concepts discussed in the next chapters, you will have increased faith. Just as this was for the Centurion and the Apostles, so it is for any believer who understands their authority given by God.

Section 2

KNOW YOUR AUTHORITY

The second section of this book explores the realms of authority of a believer. The Centurion was a man under authority and in authority. When a believer knows his position, when he knows whose authority he is under, and when he knows what authority he has been given, this is increased faith.

Few believers know the authority that is theirs in Christ. Faith is knowing this authority given to believers. The Word of God clarifies these realms of authority given to believers. Here we look to the Scriptures for understanding of the authorities we are under and are given.

Chapter 8

Beginnings of Authority

W hen did the concept of authority begin? This is the same as asking 'when did God begin?' Authority is inseparably woven in the nature of God. His being God makes Him authoritative. God's position is one of absolute authority. God exists outside of creation for He cannot create Himself. As Creator, He is fully authorized to create, sustain, remold, or destroy according to His will.

Authority Before Creation in the Trinity

Authority existed BEFORE creation and was and is present in the Trinity. Father, Son, and Holy Spirit existed before creation, apart from creation, and outside of the created order. They are three in one: one God who is Father, Son, and Holy Spirit. The triune God is one in three persons.

The main distinction between these three is primarily a difference in position and authority: God the Father is always the head; Jesus, God's Son, and the Holy Spirit are subject to the authority of God the Father. Jesus said that He can do nothing apart from His Father. He only does what He sees His Father doing. The Holy Spirit also does not speak on His own authority, but whatever He hears He speaks. So authority is a glorious thing that is present within the Triune God. The Trinity itself has order with an authority structure.

> "Jesus said to them, "Truly, truly, I say to you, the Son can do nothing of his own accord, but only what he sees the Father doing; for whatever he does, that the Son does likewise" John 5:19.

> "I can do nothing on my own authority; as I hear, I judge; and my judgment is just, because I seek not my own will but the will of him who sent me" John 5:30.

Jesus, the Son of God, though being God Himself, does not seek His own will but the will of Father God. He was obedient to God the Father unto death. Though equal with God the Father, He completely obeyed His Father. He demonstrated this glorious relationship and displayed the eternal significance of submission to authority. The Father gives authority to His Son because the Father God has that authority to give to whom He wills. "The Father judges no one, but has given all judgment to the Son" John 5:22.

Authority is present everywhere in creation and outside of creation. The acts of God issue from His throne. His throne is established on His authority. All things are created through God's authority and all physical laws of the universe are established and maintained by His authority.

Authority Provides and Protects

Authority is the very being of God the Father. His authority is compassionate, patient, loving, and fatherly. All the attributes of God are related to his authority and come forth from His authority.

Authority is God's means for protection and provision. We often misunderstand authority as something which oppresses us, hurts us, and troubles us. This is a distortion of a proper understanding of authority. God's authority is not oppressive or hurtful or troublesome. He uses authority to replenish us. His motive for authority is for protection, to bestow His riches on us, and supply needs.

We see protection and provision coming from our own parents as we grow to become adults. The whole animal kingdom also cares for and provides for their young ones. This is an innate and instinctive expression of authority. I saw my parents functioning to provide and protect throughout my childhood and beyond into adulthood.

I grew up in a small town. My brothers and I were allowed to play outside most of the day during the summer months. My parents owned a lot next door where we played many different games. There was a large tree on the corner of the lot that had numerous places to sit in the branches. One evening about six of us were sitting in the tree. The canopy of the leaves and branches provided almost complete cover. There was a small hole where the sky could be seen through the leaves. I was eating an apple at the time and wondered if I could throw it through that hole. When I mentioned it to the others, the plan evolved into a further challenge: could I throw the apple out the hole and hit a car driving on the street nearby?

As the next car came down the street, I threw the apple successfully through the small hole and waited to hear if it would hit the car. There was no such sound except the car screeched to a halt. We could see that the driver was getting out of his car. I was the first to jump out of the tree so I ran home into the garage and hid under the car. My brother came later and made it into the entry area of our home before he was caught by the driver of the car who was a senior in high school and played on the football team.

My Dad heard some commotion and came to the door. When he said, "What is going on here?" the driver let go of my brother. I came out from under the car and soon the truth also came out. The apple I had thrown did miss the car. He had his window rolled down and the apple hit him in the head. Dad was there to protect my brother and me. He was also present to provide an opportunity for me to seek forgiveness from the one I had hit. A few days later this young man returned to our home to apologize for letting his anger rule him at the time.

God has established authority on earth to extend His protection and provision. Parents and other authority positions on earth are an extension of God's authority to protect and provide for children. All delegated authorities exist for these purposes. God blessed Abraham so he could be a blessing to others. God chose the Hebrew nation to be blessed and extend God's provisions to all nations. God established order and authority in His creation in order to protect and provide for His creation. Being under authority confers great benefits for such protection and provision. It is risky to come out from under authority as this position is removed from sources of protection and provision.

Rebellion Against Authority[1]

God created order in the unseen heavenly realms with ranks of angels, seraphim, cherubim, and archangels. These rankings of angels worship and serve God in submission to His will. Each of these angelic beings knew their position in the ranks that God established. There was complete order and clarity of structure of God's delegated authority in heaven.

Then there was rebellion in the ranks of heaven. Lucifer rebelled against God's authority, wanting to be God himself. He took one third of the angels with him in this rebellion. He was cast out of heaven, away from God's presence. He lost his position and authority under God in heaven. Since then he has no authority or power except that which is given to him. God has not yet destroyed Lucifer and the demons that followed him, but cast them into hell to be kept until the judgment.[2] God allows Lucifer, also called Satan, to tempt humans. Satan acquires some measure of authority and power when humans yield to those temptations and sin against God.

Lucifer, as a serpent, tempted Eve to also rebel against God's authority. He did this by appealing to a similar desire that he himself had – to have knowledge of good and evil and be like God. Eve succumbed to this temptation. Since then all human beings have fallen short of the glory of God because we have also rebelled against his authority.

We cannot serve God by going a way of rebellion. God's grace accomplished in the work of Jesus Christ has reconciled us with God and brought us back into a relationship with Him as the Father God, bringing us back to subjection and obedience to His authority. The Centurion understood obedience to authority and Jesus called this great faith. There are two important matters: trusting God for salvation and obeying His authority, thereby declaring Jesus as Savior and Lord.

Satan is not as threatened by one proclaiming the word of Christ as compared to one who is subject to the authority of Christ. The primary controversy of the whole universe is centered on who in fact shall have the authority. Our conflict with Satan is the direct result of our attributing authority to God and obeying His word; the devil trembles at such a person.

But those who are in rebellion will lose the presence of God. Isaiah says that the Lord's hand is not shortened that it cannot save or His ear dull that He cannot hear, but our iniquities make a separation between us and God and our sins will hide His face from us.[3] Where there is rebellion and reviling among us, we will lose the presence of God. Jesus will never leave or forsake us, but when we disregard or rebel against God's authority, we leave Him and our fellowship with Him becomes distant.

Rebellion involves despising authority, choosing our own way, and resisting the will of our Father God. Rebellion is not submitting to God the Father and disobedience to His word. Jesus said the gates of Hades shall not prevail against the church.[4] Nevertheless, a rebellious spirit opens up the door whereby the enemy can establish a foothold in a person and thereby acquire a degree of ineffectiveness and control. Only the obedient can shut Hades gates and release the life that comes from God.

Countless numbers of Christians are living in a state of rebellion. They are choosing to walk on the wide path that leads to destruction. Many Christians walk a path of destruction as an outgrowth of a rebellious spirit within. The narrow path of obedience and submission to authority leads to life.

> "Enter by the narrow gate; for the gate is wide and the way is easy, that leads to destruction, and those who enter by it are many. For the gate is narrow and the way is hard, that leads to life, and those who find it are few" Matthew 7:13.

Chapter 9

Absolute and Delegated Authority

Absolute Authority

God the Father was, is, and always will be in absolute authority. He is above all beings and things, answering to no one. Everything seen and unseen is under His command. God's absolute authority existed before creation, continues through all time, and extends after the end of all things. He is eternally in charge with all things and beings subject to Him. God's authority never changes, never weakens, and never evolves.

The whole Bible is about this issue of authority. God is King and Lord. God the Father is in charge and what He says and does is without question. He does whatever He pleases because He is King of kings and Lord of lords. "For I know that the Lord is great, and that our God is above all gods. Whatever the Lord pleases he does, in heaven and on earth, in the seas and all deeps" Psalm 135:5-6.

God establishes a system of authority in order to manifest Himself. Before the visible heavens and earth were created, God created angels with clear lines of authority. There are heralding angels and warrior angels of varying positions and rank of authority. Delegated authority in the spiritual realms existed before the creation of the visible created matter. How dignified is this delegated authority in the spiritual realms. It should not be despised; any reviling of it will result in the loss of spiritual power and blessing.

Delegated Authority

In addition to heavens authority structure, God has also set up delegated authority also in the creation in which we live. There are many realms of human authority including emperors, kings, presidents, governors, deputies, chiefs, police, landlords, bosses, employers, husbands, wives, fathers and mothers. These delegated authorities are everywhere around us. There are great benefits of protection, order, and provision that God has arranged through these delegated authorities. God even authorized a whole nation, the Hebrew people of Israel, and blessed them so they could be a blessing to the whole world. We may prefer to receive benefits directly from God, the absolute authority, but almost always He provides through delegated authority.

Just as we receive blessing through God's delegated authorities when we submit to and receive from them, sinning against and rebelling against these delegated authorities is sinning against and rebelling against God Himself. This has consequences of creating separation from God Himself and the blessings and protection that comes from God through these delegated authorities.

All of these delegated human authority positions have been corrupted by the fall into sin, but this does not change God's word to us to obey them. Some of those in positions of authority have turned from their responsibilities of servant leadership to domineering over those in their charge. Abuses of this delegated power and authority are abounding. Tending and caring has been exchanged with harshness, selfish ambitions instead of generous provision, disorder in place of order, shameful gain instead of provision, injustice instead of justice, service to the leader in authority rather than being served by said leader.

Despite the shortcomings of human delegated authorities, God's word calls us to submit to those set over us. Jesus saw this submission in the Centurion and called it great faith. The Centurion said he was a man under authority. Certainly the officers set over the Centurion were flawed in some way in their execution of authority. None of the human delegated authorities are perfect in their position and execution of authority. The commandment to honor father and mother pertains to every father and mother, all of which are imperfect. Children are to obey their parents, for this pleases the Lord.[1]

> "Let every person be subject to the governing authorities. For there is no authority except from God, and those that exist have been instituted by God. Therefore he who resists the authorities resists what God has appointed, and those who resist will incur judgment" Romans 13:1.

The parable of the vineyard and the tenants focuses on delegated authority. The owner of the vineyard sent servants to the tenants to collect fruit, but the tenants rejected this delegated authority. They beat the servants and treated them shamefully. Then the owner sent his son, a delegated authority of higher position, whom they cast out of the vineyard and killed. The owner of the vineyard then came to destroy those tenants and gave the vineyard to be attended by others. The owner himself never came to the vineyard, but sent others on his behalf. The consequences due to those rejecting the owner came also by delegated authority. Submission or rejection of delegated authority is also unto the absolute authority.[2]

Submission and Obedience[3]

This matter of submission to authority is consistent throughout Scripture. The only exception is when a delegated authority demands disobedience to God. The apostles in the early church were forbidden by authorities to preach the gospel. Peter and the other apostles stated, "We must obey God rather than men" Acts 5.29. They did not disobey God in order to obey delegated authorities' edicts. This caused them to be thrown into prison. The apostles did submit to these consequences of their disobedience and trusted God who opened the prison doors. They did not obey the charge not to preach, but they did not resist, but submitted to the prison sentence.

Daniel refused to pray to the statue god of King Darius because it would have been disobedience to God. He obeyed God when the King's command was in conflict with God's word. Yet Daniel submitted to the consequences of this by going into the lion's den, trusting God for the outcome. Daniel did not obey the command to pray to the statue, but he did not resist, but submitted to the lion's den.[4]

David remained subject to Saul even after Saul lost his anointing from God. Perhaps this is the primary factor involved in David being called a man after God's own heart. To be after God's own heart is to be subject to His absolute authority and His delegated authorities. Saul was anointed by God to be King of Israel, but he disobeyed God's commandment and was rejected by God. Saul lost his anointing as King not because he stole the spoils of war, but because he spared the best of the sheep and oxen in his sacrifice to the Lord. These were his own thoughts of how he might please God, but it was in disobedience to God's orders. To obey is better than sacrifice.

Eventually David was anointed to be the King, but Saul was still in that position. David had resources and opportunities to take Saul's life and establish himself as King. Though he was anointed for this position, David did not rebel against Saul's authority over him. David waited for God to bring him to the throne. He did not attempt to accomplish God's purposes by his own ways and means. David's responsibility before God was to be subject to the delegated authority over him. Though he fled Saul's attempts at taking his life, he did not rebel or fight against Saul. David maintained God's authority, and so he was a man after God's own heart.[5]

Jesus, who was blameless and without blemish, submitted to the authorities, even unto His death. He could have made a claim for justice, but did not. Though He was reviled and suffered, He did not react with any reviling or threats. He trusted Him who judges justly.[6] He came not to abolish the law, but to fulfill it.[7] His words and deeds did not fit into some of the Jewish customs which were based on a wrong understanding of the Scriptures. This was viewed by them as disobedience to God and the law because of their wrong perceptions of who God is and what His word states.

So submission is a matter of attitude, whereas obedience is a matter of conduct. These examples were not a rebellious spirit. They still submitted to authority, but did obey God rather than men when the orders from men forced disobedience to the Word of God. When absolute authority (God) and delegated authority (humans) are in conflict, one can render submission but not obedience. Obedience is related to conduct and is relative. Submission is related to heart attitude and is absolute. God alone receives unqualified obedience without measure; obedience to humans is qualified by God's word and will. So if a delegated authority issues an order clearly contradicting God's command, he should be given submission but not obedience.

Outward willful disobedience almost always comes from an inner decision made not to submit. Difficulties in the church are less often found in matters of outward disobedience; mostly they are related to a lack of inward submission.[8]

All authority comes from God. Unless the rules and orders of human authority force disobedience to God's word, we are to obey and do so as if we are obeying God Himself, which we are. It is to our benefit to obey as unto the Lord.

> "Slaves (servants), obey in everything those who are your earthly masters, not with eyeservice, as men-pleasers, but in singleness of heart, fearing the Lord. Whatever your task, work heartily, as serving the Lord and not men, knowing that from the Lord you will receive the inheritance as your reward; you are serving the Lord Christ" Colossians 3:22-24 (parentheses mine).

> "Obey your leaders and submit to them; for they are keeping watch over your souls, as men who will have to give account. Let them do this joyfully, and not sadly, for that would be no benefit to you" Hebrews 13:17.

Chapter 10

Under Authority

The Centurion said that he was a man UNDER authority. This was what preceded his statement regarding being IN authority. First he was under authority; then he was in authority. He was a Centurion in the army and was careful to obey those in authority over him. This submission to ones IN authority over him validated, empowered, and authorized him to say to those UNDER his authority, "Go, come, or do this." We can infer that those soldiers faithfully obeyed him because he carefully obeyed his authorities.

Obedience to God's Will

God's authority is a theme throughout all of Scripture. Obedience to God's will is the greatest demand of the Bible. Jesus said in John 14.21 "he who has my commandments and keeps them, he it is who loves me, and he who loves me will be loved by my father, and I will manifest myself to him." Love of God is defined as obedience to Him. A person who says I love God but disobeys His commandments is a liar according to 1 John. The one who has God's commandments in his heart and obeys them is the one who loves him. "He who says 'I know him' but disobeys his commandments is a liar, and the truth is not in him" 1 John 2:4.

Meeting and Knowing God's authority

Before we can effectively serve God and work for Him, doing His will, we must be overturned by His authority. Specifically, we must encounter, submit to and understand the Lordship of God the Father. Before we can be an earthen vessel whereby the transcendent power of God flows through us, we must be certain of God's authority over self. This is clear in Jesus statement: "If any man would come after me, let him deny himself and take up his cross and follow me" Matthew 16:24.

Our human nature will naturally follow its own desires and passions unless it encounters the Father's love. When this occurs we simply want to obey because His love has changed our hearts. When I came to an awakening of my faith in my first year of college, God's love was poured into my heart. As a result of this, I was eager to obey Him as a response to experiencing His love. This was not motivated by fear of consequences of disobedience but simply a desire to please and obey the One who paid a great price for my salvation and who had poured His love into my heart. Then after a few weeks of a 'honeymoon' of sorts in my relationship with the Father, I was disheartened to realize that my old sinful nature and its desires continued in me. Though redeemed by the blood of Jesus, I was yet a sinner in need of grace. This is an internal struggle that continues in every believer. The single most effective way for each of us to want to obey the Lord is by an initial encounter and regular daily encounters with the love of God. It's God's mercy and kindness that best leads us to repentance.

> "I write this to you so that you may not sin; but if anyone does sin, we have an advocate with the Father, Jesus Christ the righteous; and he is the expiation for our sins, and not for ours only but also for the sins of the whole world" 1 John 2.1-2.

Whether a person has met God's authority can be seen by that person's words and actions. Such a person understands that his own way does not work for God's kingdom. This person recognizes the authority and primacy of God's word and takes efforts to lay up God's word in his heart. Whether a person has met authority can be discerned by whether he has any rebellious words or actions and whether he reasons before God. A person who knows authority will naturally try to find authority and come under it wherever he goes, because of the protection and provision therein. A person who has contacted authority guards his tongue, is slow to speak, and quick to hear, is restrained by the fear of the Lord, and submits to His word. A person who has touched God's absolute authority is sensitive to each act of lawlessness and rebellion around him.[1] One who is under God's authority does not seek his own glory, but seeks to glorify God. "He who speaks on his own authority seeks his own glory; but he who seeks the glory of him who sent him is true; and in him there is no falsehood" John 7:18.

Under the Authority of God's Word

One who knows the authority of God and His Word would never consider adding a syllable to His Word. This is the fear of the Lord and the beginning of wisdom. God's Word is eternal. Heaven and earth will pass away, but not God's word. The eternal Word of God will not pass away.

From the very beginning of recorded history, the primacy of God's word and will is established. When Eve was tempted by the serpent, the devil, she quoted God's word to the tempter, but she added "neither shall ye touch it" to God's Word. Compare God's word to Adam in Genesis 2:16-17 with Eve's quote of it in Genesis 3:3.

> God's directive to Adam in Genesis 2:16-17: "And the Lord God commanded the man, saying, 'You may freely eat of every tree of the garden; but of the tree of knowledge of good and evil you shall not eat, for in the day that you eat of it you shall die.'"

> Eve's rendition in Genesis 3:3: "but God said, 'You shall not eat of the fruit of the tree which is in the midst of the garden, neither shall you touch it, lest

you die.'" Eve added the underlined words indicating a misunderstanding of God's word and at least some disregard of the authority of God's word.

Note the evidence of God's order and delegated authority that He established with Adam and Eve. God spoke His word regarding the tree to Adam. God did not speak directly to Eve about this tree. Actually, Eve had not yet been created. God spoke to Adam, leaving him responsible to instruct, protect, and provide for Eve, his helpmate. The same responsibility to accurately teach God's word to others, especially our offspring, is given to each of us. As God spoke to Adam and created Eve, so each 'adam' since has responsibility to instruct the 'eve' God gives us.

Eve did not accurately understand God's word spoken to Adam. She added her own words: 'neither shall you touch it.' The serpent was wise enough to go to Eve to tempt her as she did not adequately understand and submit to God's word. Adam, who heard God's word directly regarding the tree, also ate of it in disobedience and rebellion to God's command. Both Adam and Eve dismissed, disobeyed, and rebelled against God's word.

Then, after they ate of the tree of knowledge of good and evil, God spoke to Adam first regarding his sin. God followed His established order of authority by going first to Adam, not Eve. Though Eve sinned first, God went to Adam. He went to Adam as the one He had established as His authority to provide for, protect, and instruct Eve. This is how a CEO would function in a corporation. He will go to the supervisor of a department regarding issues in that department. A general in the army will go to the next in command with questions or assignments relevant to that position.

Adam's response to God was an attempt to shift blame. "The man said, 'The woman whom thou gavest to be with me, she gave me fruit of the tree, and I ate.'" Genesis 3:12. Adam admitted that he ate the fruit, but prefaced it as coming from the woman God gave him. How quickly a rebellious heart will blame the one in authority. Eve's response to God was also similar: "The woman said, 'The serpent beguiled me, and I ate.'" Genesis 3:13. Eve admitted she ate the fruit and attributed her actions to the serpent's falsehoods and discrediting of God's word. Eve's reply did not include a statement of how she herself had discredited God's word.

Since then God's Word has been discredited, ignored, explained away, redefined, reworked, disbelieved, forsaken, misunderstood, tampered with, and reinterpreted. All of this is directly connected to rebellion and human reasoning.

Knowledge of Good and Evil

When Adam and Eve ate of the tree of knowledge of good and evil, they did acquire that knowledge of good and evil. Thereafter, human reasoning is a way that seems right, but in the end it leads to death.[2] So our reasonings come from this skewed knowledge of good and evil. Such reasonings come from rebellion and rejection of authority. The human mind must therefore be transformed, renewed and restored. This is not accomplished by more human reasoning. It is an ongoing process throughout life that is directed, empowered, and inspired by the Holy Spirit and the Word of God. It is a gift from God that comes through salvation and submission of our bodies to God as a living sacrifice. This renewal and transformation of our minds is a work of God in believers that He will bring to completion at the day of Jesus Christ.

> "I appeal to you therefore, brethren, by the mercies of God, to present your bodies as a living sacrifice, holy and acceptable to God, which is your spiritual worship. Do not be conformed to this world but be transformed by the renewal of your mind, that you may prove what is the will of God, what is good and acceptable and perfect" Romans 12:1-2.

All who easily change God's word, either by adding or deleting, give evidence that they do not know authority. So they are untaught and rebellious.[3]

> Colossians 1.28-29: Him we proclaim, warning every man and teaching every man in all wisdom, that we

81

may present every man mature in Christ. For this I toil, striving with all the energy which he mightily inspires within me.

Adam and Eve's disobedience to God produced a knowledge of good and evil, that is, a human reasoning that brings its own sense of right and wrong. Since the fall of Adam, disorder has prevailed. Everyone thinks he is able to distinguish good from evil. So such reasoning is the first cause of rebellion. The serpent reasoned with Eve; Eve reasoned with Adam. Such reasoning brought forth a way that seemed right and good, but in the end it brought forth death.

There are many who have a perception of what the Bible says, but have never read it. Others read the Scriptures but are inwardly skeptical and are sifting God's word to adhere to what is likable, but discarding other words. This is a form of arguing with God, implying that God needs to get our consent for all He says and does. Man likes to build reasons as strongholds around his thought, yet these reasons must be destroyed and these thoughts taken captive to obey Christ. Man's habit of reasoning is so serious that it cannot be resolved without a battle. Paul did not use reason to fight against reason.

"For though we live in the world, we do not wage war as the world does. The weapons of our warfare are not of this world, but divinely powerful for the destruction of strongholds. We are destroying arguments and every lofty thing raised up against the knowledge of God, and we are taking captive every thought to the obedience of Christ. And we will be ready to punish every act of disobedience, once your obedience is complete" 2 Corinthians 10:3-6.

If anyone wishes to learn obedience, he must subject his own reasoning to God's will and Word. Either we live by God's authority or by human reason; it is impossible to live by both. Nevertheless God's wisdom is not unreasonable. James' epistle says that wisdom from above is open to reason. God's wisdom comes from the fear of the Lord, not from human reasoning. "The fear of the Lord is the

beginning of wisdom, and knowledge of the Holy One is insight"
Proverbs 9:10. The way to know God is through obedience. All who
live in their own reasonings have not known Him.[4]

> "By this we may be sure that we know Him, if we keep
> his commandments. He who says, 'I know Him,' but
> disobeys his commandments is a liar and the truth is
> not in Him" 1 John 2:3-4.

Our sinful rebellious nature makes it impossible for us to obey
God. We need a Savior who not only forgives us of sin, but empowers
us to obey God. Redemption brings us back to finding right and
wrong from God and His word. One who is subject to authority lives
under authority and not under reason. So what will govern our lives?
Reason or Authority. When we subject our mind, will, and emotions
to God and His word, then we acquire the beginnings of wisdom
from God. This wisdom from above is most reasonable, but does not
conform to the world's reasonings.

Chapter 11

In Authority

When Jesus instructed His apostles about increased faith, He spoke about two directions of obedience to authority. We have just discussed one of these – being under authority. The other direction of obedience comes from being in authority and accurately knowing the jurisdiction of that authority.

Authority Comes From God

All authority comes from God. "For there is no authority except from God, and those that exist have been instituted by God" Romans 13:1. We cannot successfully acquire our own authority apart from God's assignment of authority. When a police officer is promoted and authorized to serve in a certain position, though this appointment comes by other people who are authorized to do so, this authority is coming from God who institutes all authority. A Pastor is called to serve a church by the worshipping body of believers, but the authority to do so comes from God. So one who has met God's authority will not try to establish his own authority; it is established by God. A husband should not say to his wife, "I am God's established authority, therefore you must listen to me." The elders of a church need not say, "We are God's appointed authority."

He who is faithful in little will be set over much. Our part is faithfulness, especially in the little things. A student, who is faithful to complete requirements for a degree, gains qualifications for certain jobs. Faithful, honest service at a place of employment can bring an appointment to a position of higher authority. This appointment comes from God who works through the delegated human authorities.

The best and proper expression of authority comes from ones who have learned to submit to those in authority over them, especially the direct authority of God Himself. A person who has not learned obedience and has not learned to be under authority is not fit to be in authority. The great faith of the Centurion, who was UNDER authority, enabled, authorized, and empowered him to speak to those under his authority. Those under his authority obeyed him, just as the Centurion submitted to and obeyed those set over him.

The faith of the Centurion, which was not seen elsewhere by Jesus in all Israel, consisted of these components: he was UNDER authority; he was IN authority; he knew Jesus had authority to speak a word at a distance to heal his servant.

The Authority of the Believer

No one person has authority over everything and everyone. Each person occupies various positions under and in certain authority structures. These vary and fluctuate throughout life as assignments to authority positions may come and go. Some people have authority over other people at a workplace; others do not. Some people have lots of possessions under their keep while others do not.

Ones who believe in Jesus Christ become ambassadors for Him. As such there is commensurate authority given by God to carry out the duties involved. "We are ambassadors for Christ, God making his appeal through us" 2 Corinthians 5:20.

The Word of God outlines some general and other specific authorities given to believers. The remaining chapters of this section clarify the authority given to believers. Understanding the authority given to believers causes increased faith.

Chapter 12

Creation Speaks To Us

The amazing detail of the created world we live in is easily perceived. Though no study is required, anyone who has learned
the basics of the sciences of Biology, Chemistry, and Physics has
acquired some of what is currently understood of the incredible
order and interconnectedness of our world and the universe. We
have acquired many tools which have given us loads of information.
A medical student learns in minute detail the makeup of DNA, the
living cell, how organs function, etc. A physicist understands some
of the physical laws of our world involving mass, time, velocity, and
energy. We understand some about the makeup of matter including
atoms and molecules.

Despite an exponential increase in the past few decades of such
knowledge about our world and universe, the unanswered questions
still greatly outnumber what is known. Nevertheless the wonders of
creation are plain to see to everyone. No special study or qualifications are required to recognize this. Those who engage in such studies
find more and more intricate detail and order. One fact discovered
about our world often generates multiple questions that have yet to
be answered.

These incredible, indescribable wonders of our world and universe speak clearly of God the Creator. Though creation does not
itself speak with human words, its message is a resounding testament
to God the Father who, out of nothing, created what now exists, the

heavens and the earth. So no one has an excuse; each must reckon with the obvious truth that God created the heavens and the earth. Even if one has never heard the gospel message, creation itself speaks of a loving God who has created us and provides for us.

"For what can be known about God is plain to them, because God has shown it to them. Ever since the creation of the world his invisible nature, namely, his eternal power and deity, has been clearly perceived in the things that have been made. So they are without excuse" Romans 1:19-20.

Authority Over The Earth

We are not just placed in this world to dwell in it and benefit from its resources. God has given us a special position of authority and dominion. So we look to the Word of God to understand the authority given to all people and specifically to those who believe in Jesus and are adopted as children of God. Again, just knowing our position and authority in Christ brings about an increase of faith. So we are striving to know the authority we have as believers. Then we endeavor to use it appropriately for God's purposes.

In the first chapters of Genesis, we learn that God gave people dominion over the earth and all that dwells on it and in it. We were created by God and placed on earth to dwell here, to be fruitful and multiply, and to extend the blessings to others and to the earth itself. We are given a certain authority over part of creation. We have dominion given by God over the earth and all living things on it. We are not given dominion over the sun, the stars, and galaxies. There is no mention in Scripture of extraterrestrial authority or dominion. We obviously cannot attend to such galactic and intergalactic authority. We are however given a very large amount of authority here — dominion over all the earth and living things on it. Based on this assignment we can decide to dig a hole or make a hill. We can add water to the ground or set it ablaze with fire. We have authority over all other living species on earth.

"Then God said, 'Let us make man in our image, after
our likeness; and let them have dominion over the fish
of the sea, and over the birds of the air, and over the
cattle, and over all the earth, and over every creeping
thing that creeps on the earth'" Genesis 1:26.

"Thou hast given him dominion over the works of thy
hands; thou has put all things under his feet, all sheep
and oxen, and also the beasts of the field, the birds of
the air, and the fish of the sea, whatever passes along
the paths of the sea" Psalm 8:6-8.

"I have given you authority to tread upon snakes and
scorpions..." Luke 10:19.

"For every kind of beast and bird, of reptile and sea
creature, can be tamed and has been tamed by human-
kind, but no human being can tame the tongue – a
restless evil, full of deadly poison" James 3:7-8.

Humans have authority and dominion given by God to use the
resources of the earth and to care for the earth and all that dwells in
it. Authority exists for purposes of protection, provision, refreshing
and renewal. Our role of dominion over the earth and all that dwells
therein is not for exploitation, but for protection and caring. We are
free to use these abundant resources for our needs as they are provided by God for us. The earth and its resources house great amounts
of resources for food, shelter, and energy. These are ours to use and
manage, or misuse and mismanage, because we have been given
dominion over the earth and all that resides on it. As for any realm of
delegated authority, we can make wise or unwise decisions regarding
the dominion over the earth given to people.

Endless Energy

There are boundless amounts of energy available around us. We
use petroleum products, solar and wind energy, and hydroelectric

energy sources. Yet there is concern about running out of energy when our world consumes and seems to require more and more energy. What if it were true that there is enough energy in a small nail to heat your home for a year? This would be fantastic news. Most people would not believe this. We would be rid of our concern for using up our energy reserves. Well, it's not true that a small nail can heat your home for a year. The truth is there is enough energy in a small nail to heat an average size home for about 40 years!

Most people can quote Einstein's famous equation "E=mc²"; few people understand what this equation is stating. $E=mc^2$ gives us a relationship between energy, mass, and the speed of light. $E=mc^2$ is saying energy (E) is equal to the mass (m) of an object multiplied times the speed of light (c) and again multiplied times the speed of light (c). A small nail weighs about 0.7 of an ounce or 20 grams or 0.02 Kg. The speed of light is about 186,000 miles per second or 300,000,000 meters per second. So the amount of energy in a small nail is 0.02 Kg x 300,000,000 m/s x 300,000,000 m/s. This equals 1.8 x 10^{15} Kg m²/s² or 1,800,000,000,000,000 joules of energy. A huge amount of energy resides in a small nail.

This is the type of energy released when the atoms undergo a fusion reaction. The mass of the nail gets converted into energy when the atoms fuse together. The sun releases its energy by the same method. Very hot temperatures are required for this reaction to sustain itself. The temperature of the sun maintains an ongoing reaction which provides light, heat, and energy in every direction including the earth, wherever it is on its orbital path.

This type of fusion reaction has been reproduced by physicists in the laboratory, but there are yet not safe enough ways to control this type of reaction for regular use. Any object with mass has a great amount of potential energy. So there is no energy crisis with regard to the amounts of energy available to us. The challenge is how to safely harvest, manage, store, transport, and use all this energy. Authority to do so is given us by God.

As regarding the food God supplies, there is also more than enough food available to satisfy all living things. Where there is a shortage of food, it is generally not a matter of supply but one of distribution. Some of the responsibility of providing food to others is given to us as we are ones in authority for purposes of provision and protection. Yet it is God who has made the seed that contains internal potential for producing plants. Together with water, carbon dioxide, and nutrients from the earth, plants grow under the energy from the sun, producing food supplies around the world. He watches over the feeding of His creatures. "Look at the birds of the air: they neither sow nor reap nor gather into barns, and yet your heavenly Father feeds them. Are you not of more value than they?" Matthew 6:26.

Speak to Creation

Jesus demonstrated His authority over creation. "Even the wind and sea obey him," the disciples said as He calmed the storm.[1] These elements of creation obeyed Jesus when He spoke. At another time He gave orders to Peter to go to the sea and cast a hook. In the first fish that came up he found a shekel for paying the tax. This was just as Jesus told Peter it would be.[2] Jesus also spoke to the fig tree that did not bear fruit. Jesus' words caused it to wither immediately.

> "And seeing a fig tree by the wayside he went to it, and found nothing on it but leaves only. And he said to it, 'May no fruit ever come from you again!' And the fig tree withered at once. When the disciples saw it they marveled saying, 'How did the fig tree wither at once?' And Jesus answered them, 'Truly, I say to you, if you have faith and never doubt, you will not only do what has been done to the fig tree, but even if you say to this mountain, "Be taken up and cast into the sea," it will be done'" Matthew 21:19-21.

After Jesus demonstrated His authority over creation, He makes an incredible statement to His followers: with faith, and no doubting, we can move even mountains. Jesus is telling His disciples here to speak to the earth and its inhabitants. Such words spoken in faith, that is, spoken by ones who are under authority and in position of authority, just as the Centurion with great faith understood, have great power and effects.

Jesus spoke and the wind and sea, the fish, and the fig tree obeyed His words. These were parts of creation that had no ears to hear what Jesus spoke. They had no mind that could comprehend what was said. Jesus spoke to His creation as the Son of God and these parts of creation, without ability to hear and understand, obeyed Him. He instructed His disciples to do the same.

Jesus also said we should preach the gospel to the whole creation. He said to them, "Go into all the world and preach the gospel to all creation" Mark 16:15. So the good news of the gospel is to be preached to all generations, to all nations, to children and grandchildren, to parents and grandparents, to all people. More than this, the gospel is to be preached also to our dogs and cats, our property, our plants and vegetation. It is to be preached to the neighbor's dogs, cats, trees, grass, plants, and house. It is to be preached to all creation, the rocks and hills, the lakes and fields. Preach the gospel to insects, fish, and wild animals. Preach the gospel to all creation.

Creation Waits

Romans 8 says creation itself is groaning in travail, waiting for the adoption as sons, the redemption of our bodies. Creation is waiting for believers to understand and use the loving, caring authority God has given to believers.

> "For the creation waits with eager longing for the revealing of the sons of God; for the creation was subjected to futility, not of its own will but by the will of him who subjected it in hope; because the creation itself will be set free from its bondage to decay and obtain the glorious liberty of the children of God. We know that the whole creation has been groaning in travail together until now; and not only the creation, but we ourselves, who have the first fruits of the Spirit, groan inwardly as we wait for adoption as sons, the redemption of our bodies" Romans 8.19-23.

Creation yearns for the children of God to know and use their authority appropriately for protection, provision, renewal, and refreshing. Creation waits for the children of God to be revealed, for their adoption as sons, and the redemption of their bodies. Jesus knew His Sonship and functioned in that authority. Now we who believe are joint heirs with Him as we are adopted into God's family. When the adopted children of God understand their position and delegated authority given by God, their faith brings benefit to creation. Creation itself eagerly longs for this to occur.

More than this, freedom from the bondage to decay will occur at the end of time, when believers' are adopted as sons and their bodies are redeemed. Currently the whole creation is in a process of decay. The second law of thermodynamics states: entropy (disorder) is always increasing in the universe. For a time there may be increased order, but over time and looking at the universe, disorder always increases. Incidentally, this law directly conflicts with the theory of evolution which states order has increased over millions of years.

We see decay all around us. Anything 'new' will eventually lose its luster. The effects of moisture, heat, sun and wind cause weathering or decay. Over time our bodily functions, strength, agility, and reflexes decline. This process functions in creation as a result of the fall of humans into sin. Creation will someday be set free from this bondage to decay and obtain the glorious liberty of the children of God. "He who sat on the throne said, 'Behold, I make all things new'" Revelation 21:5.

Jesus tells us that with mustard seed faith we can speak to the mountain, to the mulberry tree, to the sycamine tree, fig tree etc.[3] Jesus picked these elements of creation in these Scriptures to hearken to this authority and dominion we have over the earth and all that dwells in it. Furthermore, this authority is augmented and empowered in those who believe and are filled with the Holy Spirit.

Moses struck the rock to make water flow. He did this using the rod of God that he was authorized to use. He also did this as one exercising his dominion over the earth. Water came forth from the rock for the people as Moses used the rod as God instructed him. Water came forth because God delegated authority to Moses. Moses was careful to obey the Lord God's instructions. God could have provided water directly to the people, but He gave authority and power to Moses to act on behalf of God and release God's power to attend to the thirst of the people. Had Moses not struck the rock, there would not have been water flowing from the rock. Moses knew his position and authority before God and was careful to do as the Lord instructed. Moses used the authority given to him and struck the rock.[4]

So how can you use your authority and dominion over the earth? First, you must understand your position and authority in Christ as discussed above. You may then have some certain specific authority and responsibility. If you own property it is your position to oversee and manage it. You may have ownership of plants and animals that are under your care. You can use your natural authority by protecting and providing for these things. You can use your spiritual authority by speaking directly to the elements of God's creation as you are guided by the Word of God and the Holy Spirit.

Chapter 13

Devils and Unclean Spirits

F ew Christians know their authority in Christ. Of those who know it, few are using it. We should know whose authority we are under and carefully obey. We should use wisely the authority we have been given. So we continue to acquire increased faith by understanding our position under and in authority, just as Jesus saw that the Centurion understood, calling it great faith.

The Word of God instructs us regarding our authority. We find Scriptures indicating the authority we have in the unseen world over the power of the enemy: "And he called to him his twelve disciples and gave them authority over unclean spirits, to cast them out" Matthew 10:1; "I have given you authority to tread upon snakes and scorpions, and over all the power of the enemy; and nothing shall hurt you" Luke 10:19. Believers have authority to cast out unclean spirits and believers have authority over all the power of the enemy.

The Power of the Enemy

God has authority over Satan and all of the fallen angels who followed him. God gives some, but not all, of that authority to believers. The Scriptures do not indicate that we have the same authority as God Himself does over evil spirits. Believers are given authority to cast out unclean spirits and authority over all the power of the enemy. This is not authority over the enemy himself. It is authority over all his/their power, but not the beings themselves. God retains His own authority to cast them into hell and bring them to judgment. We have authority over all the power of the enemy and are able to cast out unclean spirits in Jesus' name.

We are in a battle that wages on and on over all time. This battle will not end until the end of time when Jesus returns bringing all things under His reign. "...God did not spare the angels when they sinned, but cast them into hell and committed them to pits of nether gloom to be kept until the judgment" 2 Peter 2:4. These fallen angels have been cast out of heaven because of their rebellion. They have been cast into hell awaiting judgment.

Evil remains all around us on earth because of the depravity of the human soul and the corruption in the world because of passion. Temptations arise out of the desires of the human heart. Everyone is unable to obtain victory over sin, unless being set free by the blood of Jesus and the sanctifying work of the Holy Spirit. Additionally, the evil around us comes from the power of Satan and his demons. They have been defeated by Jesus who disarmed the principalities and powers and made a public display of them.[1] They now can gain some power when humans give them opportunity through persistent and unrepentant sin, occult involvement, ancestral bondage, and mood altering drugs and chemicals.

Discernment of Spirits

Though we should not focus on the devil and unclean spirits, we should not be unaware of their schemes. "Be babes in evil, but in thinking be mature" 1 Corinthians 14:20. The Holy Spirit gives gifts of discernment of spirits and trains followers of Jesus for effective spiritual battle.

In my senior year of college I began to have dreams at night about these spiritual battles. This went on for a couple months. I'm not one to dream very much. I usually would not remember a dream if I had one. These dreams were various life circumstances where there was some kind of struggle with temptation or personal attack. Some dreams were about a ministry encounter that seems to be unfruitful. Then in each dream in various ways it occurred to me that I was in a spiritual battle and needed to use spiritual weapons for victory. In the dreams when I used these weapons there was wonderful victory. Then the dreams stopped.

A few days after this, I was checking my mail in the centrum area of the college I was attending. A classmate, with whom I had only casual acquaintance, stood next to me. I asked her how she was doing. She said she was in the hospital and they had let her out for classes. When I asked her what was wrong, she pointed to her head. I asked her to clarify. She said she was in the psychiatric ward and she was hearing voices. I asked her if visitors were allowed and if I could pray for her. She said yes and told me where I could visit her.

That evening I went to the hospital where she was in a locked in psychiatric unit. After some casual discussion, I asked her if I could pray for her. She immediately grew uncomfortable. I reminded her of our previous conversation when she said it would be okay to visit and pray with her. She started moving away from me and soon was sitting on the bed with her knees up to her chest. I told her I cared about her and believed that God could touch her and help her. Soon she spoke in what seemed to be a different type of voice, "Don't pray." I left the room wondering if I were in trouble with any of the staff in the hospital. I was more struck with the likelihood that I was encountering a woman who was demonized.

Over the course of the next four weeks, I ministered deliverance in various encounters with this woman. My roommate and a few others were also involved at times. This was a real battle against forces of darkness. The dreams that I had were no longer occurring, but those dreams were very informative for the circumstances that I was now living out. The Holy Spirit instructed and prepared me beforehand. There were amazing things that happened that could only be explained by the presence and activity of an unseen world. This woman had participated in occult activities and thus was demonized. There were numerous occasions of attempts to drive the demons from her, but we were unsuccessful.

During this time I had a dentist appointment for a general cleaning and check up. The dentist discovered a cavity that needed to be filled. It was a small job so it was taken care of at that appointment. A few days later my tooth began to hurt badly. I returned to the dentist, but he could find nothing wrong and stated there was nothing that explained this pain. That evening I met again with this woman and casually mentioned that I was having tooth pain. Her immediate comment was, "They told me they were going to do that to you." I was shocked to hear this and dismissed it at the time because my agenda there was for her deliverance, which did not yet occur that evening. All along I had been mindful of the authority we have been given over all the power of the enemy, and nothing shall harm us. I had not thought that my tooth pain could be the result of an attack of the enemy. So I took my stand and spoke a word of command to bind and drive away whatever powers or forces or assignments causing this dental pain. The next morning I woke up with no pain.

We do not need to suspect that every trouble or calamity, discouragement or disappointment, trial or tribulation is caused by an attack of the enemy. Jesus said the trials and tribulations and temptations would come; He did not come into this world to remove them from us. When operating in the front lines of this battle for the souls and lives of people, we may encounter an occasional need for cleansing and healing. We continue to believe and hold to the truth that we have authority over these powers of darkness and they will not harm us.

We did not tell many people about ministry we were doing except for some believers that joined in prayer. One evening there was very powerful ministry occurring in our dorm room where we were again attempting to drive out the demons from her. We learned later that there was a gathering just below us of about thirty believers who are praying for us. This was not scheduled. These believers simply met and began to pray. She was not set free until the next night when I switched my strategy, refusing to contend and deal with interruptions and distractions from these demonic forces. I spoke in the name of Jesus, commanding them to be quiet so that I could speak directly to the mind, heart and soul of this woman. At once there was peace; I was able to share the gospel with this woman. Up until that time I referred to Jesus as the one to whom I pray, because saying His Name caused painful reactions in her by the demonic forces. She was afraid to speak of His Name for fear of the suffering that she had experienced. That evening I led her in prayer to call upon the name

of Jesus. I led her in words of command to drive out the evil forces
from her. She was set free and no longer hearing voices.

Bind the Strong Man

A significant number of the recorded encounters of healing in
the New Testament involved addressing some kind of power assignment or battling the forces of darkness. Jesus and His disciples did
not focus on evil spirits, but attended to this battle when needed.
Not every healing encounter involves pushing back forces of darkness, but if this battle is ignored, some will not receive deliverance
and healing.

Some people are held in physical illness or disease because of
some type of spiritual stronghold. Sometimes, but not always, there
may be a spiritual power assignment that needs to be bound or broken
and driven away before healing can occur. Though the whole world
is in the power of the evil one[2], a natural protection from these forces
of evil prevails. That is to say, demonic powers do not have the right
to completely seize, occupy, or control a person. This protection is
far stronger of course when a person is baptized and believes in the
name of Jesus. People who are demonized[3] and needing deliverance
ministry may often, but not always, have made some kind of actions,
agreements, or activities that opened the door for such a stronghold
to be established. This could be from habitual sin, occult activity and
involvement, ancestral bondage handed down through generations,
or traumatic experiences. "How can one enter a strong man's house
and plunder his goods, unless he first binds the strong man? Then
indeed he may plunder his house" Matthew 12:29.

A man came to our weekly healing meeting on Wednesday morn-
ings at my church. He walked in slowly with a walker that he had
been using for the past eighteen months. I asked him if there was
any injury event as he was a middle-aged man who would normally not need a walker. He told me that he fractured his femur, the
long bone in the upper leg. He had surgery to fixate his femur and
was not to bear weight on this leg for twelve weeks. When he was
allowed to begin rehab and weight-bearing, the bone at the frac-
ture sight had not healed. His leg crushed, the bone edges crumbled,

and his leg shortened by about two inches. Since then he had been walking with the assistance of a walker and was in constant pain with weight-bearing.

I began to minister healing to him much like any other healing encounter by first laying hands on him and asking the Holy Spirit to come and touch him. Then I spoke a word of command to his leg to grow out and become the same length as the other one. I spoke to the pain and commanded it to leave. I spoke to the weakness he was experiencing and stated 'receive your strength.' I waited for a little bit and nothing happened. I was going to move on to pray for the next person, but I stopped to consider the possibility that some type of power assignment of the enemy was holding him in this way, perhaps from the trauma of the initial injury itself.

So I stated to him that I wanted to try one other thing. I spoke a word of command to bind and drive out any stronghold or power assignment that may have attached to him at the time of his traumatic injury, holding him in this condition. Then I repeated exactly what I initially spoke by word of command for this leg to grow out in the pain and weakness to be resolved. He interrupted me at this time and stated that he could feel something. I was holding on to his ankles at the time and could see that his short leg was moving. In less than a minute his leg had grown to become the same length as the other. He immediately stood up and walked without a limp. His pain was gone. He left the walker there and walked out normally.

That next Sunday at church he came to me and asked how I prayed for him, because he had many different people pray for his healing over the past eighteen months but there were no results. I told him two important points: 1) I did not really pray, I spoke to the mountain; and 2) the first mountain I spoke to was not the right mountain. Apparently there was some type of stronghold or power assignment attached to his injury and that needed to be addressed first.

His initial injury provided an opportunity for spiritual forces from the enemy to keep him from recovery. I did not know of any particular sin that he needed to confess; I did not lead him in any prayer for forgiveness. He was held in this condition because of a battle involving unseen realms of spiritual powers. For him, it was enough to drive these powers away in the name of Jesus.

Just as a power assignment of the enemy can hold a person in illness, unconfessed sin can also hinder a person from receiving God's healing power. It is appropriate to ask if there is any matter that should be confessed to God to receive His forgiveness. Without digging for a list of sins, be very careful not to communicate any kind of accusation or condemnation. If needed, confession can be done privately and silently before God. Confession and forgiveness may be necessary in breaking down forces that hold a person in some kind of disease or infirmity.

Remember the electricity analogy. If a light bulb does not work, we do not doubt electricity. Rather we change the light bulb. If that does not fix the problem, we look at the switch or the wiring. When healing does not occur, we can consider other 'mountains', including a power assignment of the enemy or unrepentant sin. It is God's nature to heal. He paid the price for our salvation and healing on the cross. Now He's given this ministry to the church and we are growing in faith and learning to use our authority as believers to address the "circuitry" to let the light of heaven shine through us.

God's Intent for His Church

The subject of demonology is not the intent of this writing. The main concept of the believer's authority over the power of the enemy is essential for Christians. We should not be ignorant or neglectful of the battle we are in, but we should worship and focus on Jesus, not on the enemy.

When a person believes in Jesus and is baptized, the cleansing blood of Jesus brings freedom and deliverance. This person is transferred from the kingdom of darkness into the kingdom of light. This light within believers cannot be overcome by darkness. The demons understand this and tremble. Believers have protection in the waters of baptism and the blood of Jesus. The sacrament of Baptism in confessional churches includes prayers and statements of deliverance from the powers of the devil.

Besides this great protection through the blood of Jesus and the covenant of baptism, believers have authority to drive out evil spirits and over the power of the enemy. The thief comes to steal, kill and destroy, but Jesus has come to give us abundant life.[3] The church has great power and authority over these unseen forces, but seldom are they used. I believe this is a reason why churches stagnate and do not grow. Churches are holding bazaars while the devil steals, kills and destroys. The church does not know well enough their authority here. Furthermore, the church has not used the spiritual weapons of warfare available to address power assignments of the enemy.

God's intent was that the church would proclaim this manifold wisdom of God to the rulers and authorities in heavenly realms. This was His eternal purpose which He accomplished through Jesus Christ our Lord. Most people would not define the church in this way that Paul did. The purpose of the church is often defined as ones who worship God, care for others, spread His word to other people, etc. These are worthy, appropriate understandings of the purpose of the church, but the Scripture says God's eternal purpose and intent was for the church to make God's wisdom known to principalities and powers in the heavenly realms.

> "His intent was that now, through the church, the manifold wisdom of God should be made known to the rulers and authorities in the heavenly realms, according to his eternal purpose which he accomplished in Christ Jesus our Lord" Ephesians 3:10-11.

If I were the author of these words, I would have written, "…the manifold wisdom of God should be made known to non-believers so they would repent and believe in Jesus." The Scriptures clearly state here that the eternal purpose of the church is to proclaim these matters to the unseen world of principalities and powers. This happens when the church worships, when the gospel is preached, and when believers pray and recite aloud the Scriptures. This occurs when believers pray to push back the forces of darkness and to bring in revival and renewal.

We see this dynamic when Daniel prayed and waited three weeks while the angel Michael contended in heavenly realms with the prince of Persia.

"Then he continued, "Do not be afraid, Daniel. Since the first day that you set your mind to gain understanding and to humble yourself before your God, your words were heard, and I have come in response to them. But the prince of the Persian kingdom resisted me twenty-one days. Then Michael, one of the chief princes, came to help me, because I was detained there with the king of Persia. Now I have come to explain to you what will happen to your people in the future, for the vision concerns a time yet to come" Daniel 10:12-14.

Think of how different our world would be if the members of the church functioned in the authority we are given over unseen principalities and powers in the heavenly realms. This is an essential requirement for revival and awakening and a frequent "mountain" that needs moving when ministering to others.

Chapter 14

Bind and Loose

ate one evening I was returning home from a meeting at church. I opened my car door and left it open while I buckled the seatbelt. As I turned back to close the door, a woman was standing next to me and I began to feel something sharp into my ribs. She was holding a pointed scissors and began pushing it into my side. I recognized her right away as she had been attending some fellowship meetings that I was leading. She had been exhibiting some aggressive behaviors that had been escalating over the past weeks. She had previously slashed my tires on my car and threw water on me at the end of a fellowship meeting, saying "You're lucky; it was supposed to be hot water."

"I bind you," were the words that came out of my mouth without any premeditation. I had never said those words to anyone before this. The words came from my lips without any prior thought; I think they were words inspired by the Holy Spirit. Immediately she fell to the ground and lost her strength with a scissors still in her hand. A custodian was nearby, locking up the building. I called for his help and we were able to gain control of the situation.

The Keys of the Kingdom

Jesus gave to Peter the keys of the kingdom, saying "Whatever you bind on earth will be bound in heaven, and whatever you loose on earth will be loosed in heaven" Matthew 16:19. To bind is to tie up like a cattle roper ties the legs of an animal, rendering them powerless. To be bound is like a person in restraints or wearing a straight jacket. To loose is to set free like untying the legs of an animal, allowing it to run freely. Loosing removes restraints and permits freedom. To bind declares something forbidden and to loose affirms something allowed. Binding prohibits and loosing permits.

We may use the term 'bind' also for other purposes. Binding can be done to prevent risk of danger. You may bind yourself to a lifesaver before going into water. Holding a child's hand is a form of binding for protection. Additionally, the Greek term 'doulos' is translated 'slave' or 'bondservant' indicating an obligation to serve another. A bondservant is bound to serve his master. The Apostle Paul spoke of himself in this way. We also speak of the bond of marriage where vows of commitment bind a man and woman together to become one.

Human anatomy and physiology also have instances of binding. There are covalent bonds that hold molecules together. The hemoglobin molecule in red blood cells weakly binds to four molecules of oxygen. Then oxygen is 'loosed' from the hemoglobin and delivered to all parts of the body. Certain electrolyte ions and drugs are bound to proteins. These drugs, ions, or toxins that are protein bound have less impact on body receptors and metabolic functions compared with those that circulate in a free (unbound or loosed) state. Our immune system constantly surveys our bodies looking for 'non-self'. When bacteria or other foreign entities are detected by the immune system, the T cells and B helper cells bind to them and are removed.

Peter's Authority

The biblical usage of the terms 'binding' and 'loosing', come from Jesus spoken in the context of two different settings. One is when Peter, inspired by the Holy Spirit, says of Jesus that He is the Christ. Then Jesus states He will build His church and gives Peter the keys of the kingdom and authority to bind and loose. The other occurs when Jesus teaches about the process of gaining a brother who sins against another. Matthew records the first instance in chapter 16:

"Simon Peter replied, 'You are the Christ, the Son of the living God.' And Jesus answered him, 'Blessed are you, Simon Bar Jona! For flesh and blood has not revealed this to you, but my Father who is in heaven. And I tell you, you are Peter, and on this rock I will build my church, and the powers of death shall not prevail against it. I will give you the keys of the kingdom of heaven, and whatever you bind on earth shall be bound in heaven, and whatever you loose on earth shall be loosed in heaven'" Matthew 16:16-19.

"On this rock I will build my church." Note that Jesus said HE will build HIS church. He did not tell Peter to build Peter's church and John to build John's church and James to build James' church. He did not set up His disciples to compete for members in their churches. He did not delegate the task of building the church. For church leaders today, the message is the same: Jesus will build His church. There is no room for a Pastor's own agenda. There is no place in the church for selfish ambition. This leads to disorder and wrong practice. "Unless the Lord builds the house, those who build it labor in vain" Psalm 127:1.

Jesus did not delegate the process of building His church, but He did delegate certain authority here in this text. Jesus spoke specifically to Peter only. The phrases "I will give you", "whatever you bind", and "whatever you loose" in their original Greek text clarify this. Each of the three times the word "you" in this verse is used, it occurs as a singular pronoun. Each "you" is not plural, indicating that Jesus spoke to Peter specifically. Our English does not distinguish between 2nd person singular and plural pronouns. The word "you" can mean just one or more than one. In Greek there are different words for singular and plural 2nd person pronouns. These words of authority spoken by Jesus were delivered to Peter only as Jesus uses the singular pronoun as He addresses Peter. This verse occurs in the context of Jesus building His church on 'this petra' or 'this rock', making an obvious connection to Peter's name which means 'rock.'

Whatever you bind/loose on earth, will be bound/loosed in heaven. So whatever Peter bound, prohibited, or forbade in the church had divine authority. Whatever Peter loosed, permitted, or commanded in the church also had divine authority. Jesus built His church on Peter, the rock, who was to be guided by the Holy Spirit in the organization of the church. As Peter obediently followed Jesus' building of His bride, the church, Peter could use the keys of the kingdom to bind and loose. This had God's authority behind it.

Later, as recorded in the Book of the Acts of the Apostles, Peter received revelation from God regarding the message of the gospel going to the Gentiles. Peter fell into a trance and saw the heavens opened and something descending like a great sheet. In it were all kinds of animals, reptiles and birds. A voice spoke telling him to rise, kill and eat. Peter's religious custom was to never eat anything common or unclean. The Lord replied saying, "What God has cleansed, you must not call common." This vision happened three times. What was unclean by Jewish standards was now permitted by God. This was revelation of the gospel going to the Gentiles. Peter then loosed or permitted this activity. He did so because of the revelation of the Holy Spirit in the vision and because he saw the Holy Spirit poured out on Gentile believers as evidence of God's plan. Jesus was building His church on Peter, the rock. The good news was loosed to all nations.[1]

Then as the Gentiles came to faith there were some believers from Judea and other converts from the Pharisees who stated that these Gentile believers must be circumcised and keep the Law of Moses in order to be saved. The apostles and elders met in Jerusalem to consider this matter.

> "And after there had been much debate, Peter rose and said to them, 'Brethren, you know that in the early days God made choice among you, *that by my mouth the Gentiles should hear the word of the gospel and believe.* And God who knows the heart bore witness to them, giving them the Holy Spirit just as he did to us; and he made no distinction between us and them, but cleansed their hearts by faith. Now therefore why do you make trial of God by putting a yoke upon the neck of the disciples which neither our fathers nor we

have been able to bear? But we believe that we shall
be saved through the grace of the Lord Jesus, just as
they will'" Acts 15:7-11 (italics mine).

Peter's words here were then considered further and were
accepted among the apostles and elders. Circumcision was not
required of the Gentile believers. Salvation was through the grace of
Jesus Christ. Gentile believers were then instructed to abstain from
what has been sacrificed to idols, from blood, from what is strangled,
and from unchastity. Peter was using the keys of the Kingdom here,
setting forth what was required and what was to be avoided among
believers in the church. Peter followed the revelation and instructions
he received from Father God. He used his authority to bind and loose.

Believers' Authority to Bind and Loose

The other context of the use of binding and loosing is when Jesus
teaches about forgiveness as recorded in Matthew 18:

"If your brother sins against you, go and tell him his
fault, between you and him alone. If he listens to
you, you have gained your brother. But if he does not
listen, take one or two others along with you, that
every word may be confirmed by the evidence of two
or three witnesses. If he refuses to listen to them, tell
it to the church; and if he refuses to listen even to the
church, let him be to you as a Gentile and a tax col-
lector. Truly, I say to you, whatever you bind on earth
shall be bound in heaven, and whatever you loose on
earth shall be loosed in heaven. Again I say to you,
if two of you agree on earth about anything they ask,
it will be done for them by my Father in heaven. For
where two or three are gathered in my name, there am
I in the midst of them" Matthew 18:15-20.

In this text the word 'you' is plural. It was like saying, 'you all'
or 'ya'll'. Here Jesus instructs all of His followers. The authority to

bind and loose is conferred to all believers. Specifically, this authority underscores the power of forgiveness and unforgiveness. Generally, this authority applies to "whatever."

Specifically, the authority to bind and loose in matters of forgiveness and reconciliation has divine authority. "Whosoever sins you forgive, they are forgiven. Whosoever sins you retain, they are retained." If you forgive others, God will also forgive you. If you do not forgive others, God will not forgive you. The consequences of this truth are both glorious and daunting. The glorious blessings of forgiveness bring freedom, healing, and inner peace. The daunting products of unforgiveness include bondage, disease, and inner turmoil. These are matters pertaining to eternity. Whether we forgive or not has immediate consequences regarding our fellowship with God and eternal consequences regarding our inheritance in heaven.

Generally, there is a wide range of authority that Jesus gives to His disciples in these words. He says WHATEVER you bind or loose on earth will be bound or loosed in heaven. This requires wisdom and insight into the heart of God. Such authority to bind and loose must be guided by the leading of the Holy Spirit and the written words of Scripture. Yet as Jesus said these words to His disciples, He did not attach any qualifications. He simply said whatever you bind and loose on earth will be bound and loosed in heaven. As with any delegation of authority, there will be occasions of mistakes and learning. Jesus gave this authority to us to bind and loose whatever we will, knowing that we can and would likely misuse this authority and knowing that we must as always follow the Word of God and the leadings of the Holy Spirit. The words from the Lord 's Prayer are a related request for provision and guidance: 'Thy kingdom come, Thy will be done on earth as it is in heaven.'

/How to Minister in This Realm of Authority

Many times when ministering healing, I will bind the power of the specific disease or condition involved. I also consider how to release or loose health and blessing to the person receiving ministry. For example, it is appropriate to say to someone with some type of cancer, "I bind the power of those cancerous cells and I loose or release healing and blessing by the power of the Holy Spirit in the name of Jesus."

You can use this authority to bind and loose your own personal thoughts. You can bind the power of temptations to greed, lust, anger, unforgiveness, gluttony, idolatry, etc. Jesus said temptations will come, so this does not stop temptation. Nevertheless, you can declare what you will permit and refuse in your own mind by using your authority to bind and loose. And you can loose the fruit of the Spirit[2], that is, you can determine to allow the fruit coming from the Holy Spirit. You can do the same as you minister to the inner being, the mind, will, and emotions, of others.

When Jesus gave this authority, He placed no qualifications. Whatever you bind/loose on earth will be so in heaven. There are therefore endless applications of this authority to bind and loose, but this can be like shooting arrows randomly or throwing hammers at a rainbow. Instead consider what may be the root problem and listen to the Word of God and the promptings of the Holy Spirit. Being under the authority of Father God and being careful to obey Him places us in a position to be led by the Spirit in using these tools for advancing God's kingdom.

Chapter 15

Self

ew people really know the authority they have as believers in
Jesus Christ. Of the few who do accurately know their authority
in Christ, few use it. Of the few that use their authority in Christ,
some unwisely misuse it. We should know our authority in Christ and
thereby have increased faith. We should use it wisely for purposes of
advancing God's kingdom.

The next area of authority we should explore is authority over
self. At first thought this may seem obvious. We all make our own
decisions — what we will say and do, where we will spend our time
and resources. Do we really make all of these decisions and have this
authority over self? There are so many aspects of life that are prescribed for us. We are told what to do by governing laws, employers,
friends and family. With duties, bills to pay, and obligations, it can
appear that we really make relatively few decisions for ourselves.
What is this authority over self as described in Scripture?

An Inner Struggle

Every human has an inner struggle. We can know what is right
to do or say and yet be tempted to do the opposite. When a temptation appeals to an inner desire, an inner struggle ensues. Sometimes
we feel completely powerless in this inner turmoil. An addiction to

anything typifies this battle. Every human being has fallen under the clutches of sin and its consequences.

> "For I know that nothing good dwells within me, that is, in my flesh. I can will what is right, but I cannot do it. For I do not do the good I want, but the evil I do not want is what I do. Now if I do what I do not want, it is no longer I that do it, but sin which dwells within me. So I find it to be a law that when I want to do right, evil lies close at hand. For I delight in the law of God, in my inmost self, but I see in my members another law at war with the law of my mind and making me captive to the law of sin which dwells in my members" Romans 7:18-23.

The captivity, due to this law of sin dwelling in our members, is bondage, not freedom. It is self out of control; not self in control. It is self being unable to submit to authority. Then we become slaves to whatever we obey.

> "Don't you know that when you offer yourselves to someone as obedient slaves, you are slaves of the one you obey—whether you are slaves to sin, which leads to death, or to obedience, which leads to righteousness? But thanks be to God that, though you used to be slaves to sin, you have come to obey from your heart the pattern of teaching that has now claimed your allegiance. You have been set free from sin and have become slaves to righteousness" Romans 6:16-18.

This struggle can intensify when a person believes in Jesus. This occurs because a believer is now no longer under the power of the evil one and has been born anew to a life in the Spirit of God. The old sinful nature yet continues in believers and is vulnerable to temptation and wrongdoing.

Additionally, one who is no longer under the power of the evil one now has him as an enemy. So the accuser of the brethren, the devil, hurls accusations at those who follow Jesus. Satan and his demons have not yet met their final demise which God will bring on the day of judgment. The Son of man came to destroy the works of the devil. He accomplished this task, but the devil himself awaits his final judgement from God. Meanwhile, he and his demons have some degree of power to promote evil in the world through humans who carry out their agenda.

The Solution for Self

The problems of the world are not solved by more education. We have never been more educated. Though we may have more sophisticated terms to describe humanity, though we understand more about physics, geology, chemistry, psychology, and biology, our basic problems continue. There is no evidence of decreased evil in the world because of the overall increase of knowledge in the world. Nor will government be able to pass laws or provide true solutions. We have more laws in this country than any other time. Lawmakers pass thousands of laws each year without any change in basic human nature and conditions.

The real problem is rooted in the self in need of a Savior. It is a spiritual problem requiring a spiritual remedy. The sinful nature of humans runs throughout our being and cannot be corrected except by crucifixion with Christ and living by faith in Him. This is not just the crucifixion OF Christ that brings our victory. It is our crucifixion WITH Christ that brings death to our sinful nature and resurrection life as we live by faith. Jesus not only died for us, we died with Him. Jesus died for us to pay the penalty of sin and satisfy God's righteous demand. This payment made by Jesus on our behalf brings eternal life in heaven for those who believe in Him. More than this, we died with Him on the cross to gain victory over our sinful nature. Self is properly remedied from its sinful nature only by death. Believers have been crucified with Christ. We died with Him. Those who so identify with Christ's death may also share in the power of His resurrection.

When you try to save your life, you will lose it. When you lose your life for Jesus' sake, then your life is saved.[1] When you deny self, then you gain self-control. When you die to self, being crucified with Christ, you gain newness of life.[2] When you count yourself dead to sin and alive to God, you are no longer slaves to sin.[3] When you set your minds on things that are above and not on earthly things, then you are aware of your being raised with Christ and seated with Him in heavenly places.[4] God's answer to self is crucifixion. Then the Spirit of God gives self-control.

One who has been crucified with Christ is dead to self and then seeking to do God's will by the power of the Holy Spirit. Sufferings in this life can make one either bitter or better. The Scripture exhorts rejoicing in sufferings because through them strength is acquired to live by the will of God.

> "More than that, we rejoice in our sufferings, knowing that suffering produces endurance, and endurance produces character, and character produces hope, and hope does not disappoint us, because God's love has been poured into our hearts through the Holy Spirit which has been given to us" Romans 5:3-5.

> "Since therefore Christ suffered in the flesh, arm yourselves with the same thought, for whoever has suffered in the flesh has ceased from sin, so as to live for the rest of the time no longer by human passion, but by the will of God" 1 Peter 4:1-2.

A Spirit-filled, Spirit-led life is one with self-control. Self-control is not acquired by making more firm decisions for yourself. Self-control is not a product of effectively managing your surroundings. True self-control is only acquired by yielding control to the Holy Spirit. "The fruit of the Spirit is ... self-control" Galatians 5.22,26. Self-control comes from the Holy Spirit. Self-control is not completed by using human tools such as increased resolve and dedication. We are slaves to the old nature until we are redeemed and set free by the blood of Jesus and count ourselves as ones crucified with Christ. We can choose to become enslaved again by obedience to the old nature or choose to be free and acquire self-control by obedience (faith) to the Lord.

So what does the self consist of? What specific control does the fruit of the Spirit self-control include? We are one being, made up of body, soul, and spirit. The authority of self-control is over self: body, soul, and spirit.

Body

Self-control includes your own body. There are many normal functions of the human body that are automatic, requiring no conscious effort or thought. Other processes are volitional responding to commands from the individual. The normal functions of the body which we employ every day are nothing short of incredible. Think of the amazing amount of coordination required to do normal regular activities. The arm moves immediately and automatically when commanded by the central nervous system. When walking with just two legs, unlike most other species of creation who ambulate on four or more appendages, each step with just two legs brings us to the verge of falling. Instead nerves and muscle groups are engaged by the central nervous system to bring about a very fluid efficient ambulation which hardly requires any conscious concentration.

A choir of singers can hear a pitch and remember it without humming the pitch. Then at the command of the director the choir begins the first notes of a song in beautiful harmony. Some people have what is called 'perfect pitch', an ability to hear or sing a note and detect what note sounded forth.

Each breath taken in to our lungs brings the air past about twenty divisions of the respiratory tree to the bronchioles and alveoli where gas exchange occurs. If you could spread out this area where gases interface with capillary vessels, it would cover approximately 70 square meters, about the size of a tennis court. Furthermore, each breath is warmed to body temperature and 100% humidity by the time it reaches the alveoli. So whether you are breathing the hot dry air at 110F or cold dry air at -50F, the result is the same for each breath. This is too incredible to be attributed to some accidental process of evolution. These kind of amazing functions of the human body are abundant.

Many of these bodily functions are automatic, occurring without any conscious effort. The volitional motor functions of the body do require direction and impulse from a person's will mediated through the central nervous system. These bodily functions come under the command of its head. Even in the disease states of a seizure or stroke, the body still follows the commands coming from the head. In these diseases the problems arise from the central nervous system itself.

The relationship of the body with the head, how the body immediately obeys the directions coming from the central nervous system, demonstrates the relationships of the church with her Head, Jesus Christ.[5] Each part of the church body functions in obedience to the Head of the church.

Self-control of your body is demonstrated by how you care for yourself, where you go, what you eat, and how active you are. We are given authority over our own body. So we are free to use the functions of our body as desired. We have authority over the automatic and volitional functions of our body. In Christ we have self-control as a fruit of the Holy Spirit. When we couple this authority over our own bodies with the authority we are given over every disease and every infirmity, we can thus speak a word of command to 'this mountain', in this case, our body, to minister healing to our own body where it may need healing.

Soul

Self-control includes your soul. A human soul consists of mind, will, and emotions.

Our society places a lot of value to a person's feelings and emotions. News reporters are looking for footage that shows lots of emotion. Those interviewed are often asked how they feel. Lots of attention is directed toward avoiding undesirable feelings in ourselves and others. Businesses arrange for hours of sensitivity training to avoid offending the feelings of other co-workers and patrons. There are lawsuits that claim financial payment for emotional duress.

It can appear at times that emotions are more important than the facts, the truth.

Certain circumstances can immediately trigger undesired emotions of hurt and anger that can control us. These can arise from previous unhealed wounds to one's heart and spirit or these may be an indicator of a belief system that has strayed from the truth of the Word of God. The Word of God acknowledges feelings and emotions, but does not exalt them above obedience and self-control. There are Psalms of lament where we can join with David in his prayers to the Lord expressing various emotions. David brought his emotions to the Lord in psalms and songs while he was careful to submit to authority and rejoice in the Lord his deliverer.

Throughout the Scriptures the place for emotions is clearly subject to a person's will. We are instructed to rejoice always, to put on the garment of praise for the spirit of heaviness, to weep with those who weep and rejoice with those rejoicing. We can do so because we can choose this. We can do so because we can have emotions yet not be ruled by them. We can acknowledge our emotions without becoming a slave to them. We can put on attitudes that control emotions. This is part of the self-control that comes as a fruit of the Holy Spirit.

Thoughts

Self-control also includes jurisdiction over the battleground of our thoughts. A clear understanding of the authority believers possess over thoughts is a discussion that occurs in the next chapter.

Spirit

Self-control also includes your spirit. God has made a spirit to dwell in us. "He yearns jealously over the spirit which he has made to dwell in us" James 4:5. The human spirit is the innermost being. It is begotten by God and exists for eternity. We see reference to this spirit when Jesus raised Lazarus from the dead. When Jesus said, "Lazarus, come forth," his spirit returned to him and then he came out of the tomb. During the four days he was dead, his spirit had left his body.[6] Many testimonies exist of ones who describe death or near death experiences involving their spirit leaving their body and returning. This is the human spirit that lives after the body perishes. The spirit that God made to dwell in us is eternal.

Some nurses at the hospital where I work tell of such an experience. A couple decades ago there was a man who came in by ambulance as he was in cardiac arrest. On arrival he was unconscious as his heart was not pumping blood. The doctors and nurses continued cardiopulmonary resuscitation (CPR) for almost an hour, then his heart restarted but he remained unconscious until the next morning. When the nurses returned the next day to check on him, he knew the names of each one. He had never met any of them before this. He said that he was looking down at himself and the medical team as they were attempting to revive him. He learned the names of each one because he could read the name tags. The nurses state there was no other way for him to know their names.

This spirit that God made to dwell in us is the part of us that understands our own thoughts. "For what person knows a man's thoughts except the spirit of the man which is in him? So also no one comprehends the thoughts of God except the Spirit of God" 1 Corinthians 2.11. It is the spirit of a person that understands his thoughts. No one else can comprehend the thoughts of a person except the spirit of that person. We have trouble understanding others at times even though we may live in the same culture, use the same language, even live in the same family. The human spirit is the core of an individual.

God has given each one charge over his own spirit. Paul states in his instructions regarding spiritual gifts: "The spirit of the prophets is subject to the prophets" 1 Corinthians 14:32. To be subject to something is to be under its authority. This verse states specifically that a person with prophetic gifts will receive inspiration from the Holy Spirit, but yet retains control over how and when and if those gifts will be expressed. This verse also confirms more generally that the spirit of a believer is subject to that believer. This is part of the fruit of self-control that the Holy Spirit releases in believers.

Also in that same chapter Paul states, "I will pray with the spirit and I will pray with the mind also; I will sing with the spirit and I will sing with the mind also" 1 Corinthians 14:15. In this verse the words

'I will' further establish the authority of the will of a person over his spirit (and his mind). The fruit of self-control is a Spirit-empowered governing of one's own body, soul, and spirit.

One of the fruits of the Spirit is self-control. When a Christian is empowered and baptized by the Holy Spirit, there is not a loss of control, rather a gain of self-control. Some people have a perception about the gifts of the Spirit, especially speaking in tongues, that such people are making ecstatic utterances as ones out of control. "Ecstatic" (Ek – out of; Stasis – stance or position) means "out of control". How then could it be that one of the gifts of the Spirit, speaking in tongues, is at odds with one of the fruit of the same Spirit, self-control? Actually a person gains self-control when walking in the Spirit. When one speaks in tongues, though the mind is unfruitful and not understanding what is spoken, that person's spirit prays. This person gains self-control. The gifts of the Spirit function best in a believer with self-control, a fruit of the Spirit. When we yield to the Spirit of God, we gain victory in this battle over our old nature.

Chapter 16

Every Thought Captive

———————◆———————

Believers are given authority over thoughts. We have control over what we think. Yes, you can control your thoughts. Every day we are processing many decisions in our minds. We control our thought process when walking down an aisle in the grocery store to decide which peanut butter brand to purchase. We can be careful to select from various thoughts when responding to questions at a job interview. We choose to keep certain thoughts and reject others because we have authority over our thoughts. The Scriptures give us advice about what to think.

> "Finally, brothers and sisters, whatever is true, what-
> ever is noble, whatever is right, whatever is pure,
> whatever is lovely, whatever is admirable, if anything
> is excellent or praiseworthy—think about such things"
> Philippians 4:8.

We possess an amazing God-given ability to make choices considering input from rational or irrational thinking, emotions, past experiences, others' advice, and most importantly, Scripture. "For God did not give us a spirit of timidity but a spirit of power and love and self-control" 2 Timothy 1:7. Other translations translate 'self-control' as 'a sound mind'.[1] The Holy Spirit restores self-control and a sound mind in the life of a believer. When a person submits to the Lordship of Jesus Christ, repenting of sin, denying himself, taking up his cross, and following Jesus, God gives power through the Holy Spirit to enable obedience to Him. God restores self-control to enable obedience to Jesus Christ and His Word. This includes our thoughts, the battleground where temptations and deception arise and the place where God reveals truth.

A Transformed Mind

> "Do not be conformed to this world but be transformed by the renewal of your mind, that you may prove what is the will of God, what is good and acceptable and perfect" Romans 12:2.

Our thoughts have been distorted by sin. Our thoughts need to be transformed by the Word of God and the work of the Holy Spirit. Proverbs 3:5 says "Trust in the Lord with all your heart and do not rely on your own insight." The realm of the human mind is truly a battleground. The crux of the battle resides here. The old nature at war with our new nature takes place primarily in our minds, our thinking. Temptation arises as a thought that has an appeal.

> "Let no one say when he is tempted, "I am tempted by God"; for God cannot be tempted with evil and he himself tempts no one; but each person is tempted when he is lured and enticed by his own desire. Then desire when it has conceived gives birth to sin; and sin when it is full grown brings forth death" James 1:13-15.

The human mind is also the target whereby a flaming dart from the evil one can attempt to occupy space or to give birth to sin. In addition to our own desires that can wage war in our souls, the enemy may shoot flaming darts at our thinking.[2] Those are not our thoughts unless we accept them and invest in them. Continued investment in such thoughts can eventually affect the heart or spirit of a person. We are instructed to guard our heart with all diligence, for from it flow the springs of life.[3] We are taught to set our minds on things above, not on things that are on earth.[4]

God has given us a spirit of power and love and self-control. So He has given us authority over ourselves. It may seem obvious that any person, by virtue of being human, makes his own choices and has his own authority. But the consequences of sin bring us into slavery to sin and loss of self-control. Too many Christians are not aware of the God given authority of self-control and continue as slaves to various expressions of disobedience and bondage.

> "I do not understand my own actions. For I do not do what I want, but I do the very thing I hate…For I do not do the good I want, but the evil I do not want is what I do… For I delight in the law of God, in my inmost self, but I see in my members another law at war with the law of my mind and making me captive to the law of sin which dwells in my members" Romans 7:15, 19, 22-23.

Many cannot seem to gain proper control over some parts of life and conduct. Some want others to control their lives. Some let others control them. God's Spirit is given to restore self-control.

The Weapons of Our Warfare

This is not a simple matter of making a different choice in day by day decisions. It is not like choosing between different brands of cereal or a flavor of coffee at the grocery store. Obedience or disobedience to Jesus Christ and His word has eternal consequences. This is the focus of an epic spiritual battle. We are given weapons that are divinely powerful for the destruction of fortresses. Paul viewed this as a spiritual matter requiring spiritual weapons. Our thoughts are not completely controllable by reason, study, knowledge, or a strong will. This is not a fleshly battle; it cannot be won by human tools.

> "For though we walk in the flesh, we do not war according to the flesh, for the weapons of our warfare

are not of the flesh, but divinely powerful for the
destruction of fortresses. *We are* destroying speculations and every lofty thing raised up against the
knowledge of God, and *we are* taking every thought
captive to the obedience of Christ, and we are ready
to punish all disobedience, whenever your obedience
is complete" 2 Corinthians 10:3-5 (Italics mine).

Paul said we are to wage war with divinely powerful weapons
against every lofty thing raised up against the knowledge of God. We
are to take every thought captive to obey Jesus Christ. This is evidence of the authority we have over thoughts. We are able to destroy
speculations, to conquer premature conclusions based on guessing
or hearsay, and to bring down arguments that are not founded on the
truth of God's word. We do this not by argument or persuasion, but
by using spiritual weapons with our spiritual authority.

Our mind is the primary battleground. Thoughts in the human
mind come from several sources: self, others, the devil, and the Holy
Spirit. The human mind is like a field where both wheat and weeds
coexist. First, we can generate our own thoughts and opinions. We
can have our own rationale, our own reasonings, and our own belief
system that can be based on truth or error, raised up for or against
the knowledge of God. Secondly, there are others that influence our
thoughts. Some of this is proper and beneficial as no one of us has all
insight and knowledge. Some opinions from others, however, should
be rejected. Thirdly, our mind is where the flaming darts of the evil
one are hurled. Our thoughts can succumb to the deceptions and
wiles of the enemy. God said to Cain as he struggled with temptation, "Sin is crouching at the door; its desire is for you, but you must
master it" Genesis 4:7. And lastly, our minds can also be inspired
by the Holy Spirit. God pours his love into our hearts by the Holy
Spirit and usually bypasses the mind initially. When our hearts have
encountered the living God and His love, then our minds are enlight-
ened by the Spirit of God.

This battleground requires spiritual weapons. Arguments that contend with the Word of God are like fortresses that are to be destroyed.
They are destroyed with powerful weapons that are not of the flesh

but are divine, spiritual. Paul is not referring to just some of the more important arguments and thoughts. He says EVERY lofty thing and EVERY thought are the focus of this battle.

Every Thought

This Scripture does not specify whose thoughts are to be taken captive to the obedience of Christ. Certainly Paul refers to his own thoughts. Certainly each of us has our own thoughts that we must manage. Paul used spiritual weapons to attend to the battle in his own mind. We should also use these weapons to attend to our own battles. Paul does not, however, limit this battle to his own thoughts. He also addresses the thoughts and lofty arguments of others. He was destroying speculations and EVERY lofty thing raised up against the knowledge of God. He took EVERY thought captive to obey Jesus Christ. So Paul says he used spiritual weapons also to destroy other's lofty arguments against the knowledge of God. He took other's thoughts captive to obey Christ.

His responsibility and authority to wage this battle was increased by virtue of his calling as an apostle, but he also calls every believer to engage in this battle. Paul speaks here in plural. WE do not wage war against the flesh. The weapons of OUR warfare... WE are destroying speculations... WE are taking every thought captive...

This is not some kind of mystical thought control mechanism whereby we can pretend to control another's thoughts. This is not a tool for manipulating others. It is, however, a set of tools for attending to our own thoughts in particular. It is also a description of weapons used to take other's thoughts captive to obey Christ. These are not tools to bring others thoughts to obey you or someone else. It is bringing every thought and argument to be subject to the Word of God and to obedience to Jesus Christ. It is recognizing that the human mind is a battleground requiring spiritual weapons. Paul understands that the unspiritual person is unable to receive the things of the Spirit. A battle is required to call down strongholds that hold a person who is without understanding and without seeing. "In their case the god of this world has blinded the minds of unbelievers, to keep them from seeing the light of the gospel of the glory of Christ, who is the likeness of God" 2 Corinthians 4:4.

The minds of unbelievers are blinded by the god of this world. "We know that we are of God, and the whole world is in the power of the evil one" 1 John 5:19. Unbelievers are blinded and thus cannot see the light of the gospel. Spirit-filled believers are given authority and weapons to drive away those blinders. This is an essential and powerful tool for evangelizing unbelievers. The minds of unbelievers are unable to see the good news of the gospel as they are held in the power of the evil one.

I worked at a Bible Camp for a couple summers during my college years. During this time, we took a bus load of youth to a conference in Kansas City. On the long ride back I picked up conversation with a fifteen year old girl. I was hoping to lead her to faith in Jesus Christ if she was not yet a Christian. I repeatedly steered the conversation to a point where I asked her if she understood the good news and would like to place her faith in Jesus. Each time she was silent for about a minute, then changed the subject of the conversation and evaded an answer. This went on and on for four hours.

We had an overnight stop about half way home. That night I prayed for her (not with her), remembering that the god of this world is blinding the minds of unbelievers. I used spiritual weapons of warfare to call down this power assignment over her. The next day she came to me saying that she was thinking the last evening about what was said on the bus ride. It made sense to her and she wanted to invite Jesus into her heart for forgiveness of sins and salvation. I led her in a prayer to accept Jesus as her Savior and Lord.

Enter the Kingdom Violently

"The law and the prophets were until John, since then the good news of the kingdom of God is preached, and every one enters it violently" Luke 16:16. No one enters the Kingdom of God peacefully. There is always a battle in the heavenly realms. Every person who sincerely places faith in Jesus Christ does so in the midst of a spiritual battle. The battleground is the mind and heart of the person. Spirit filled believers must attend to this battle for effective evangelism. We must use spiritual weapons that are divinely powerful for the destruction of fortresses, to remove blinds from the eyes of unbelievers, to call down arguments raised up against the knowledge of God, and take every thought captive to the obedience of Jesus Christ.

After coming into my own awakening in faith in Jesus Christ, I was concerned about my paternal grandparents' salvation. I was unsure of their readiness to meet the Lord. Every time I came home I visited them, hoping to bring them into assurance of salvation through Jesus Christ. These conversations proceeded for about a year, but there was no harvest. I was hoping that seeds of the Word were planted. I had conversation with my aunt about the dead end I was repeatedly encountering with them. She reminded me that my grandfather had been involved in the Free Masons and I should take this matter to prayer. So I used these spiritual weapons for calling down strongholds over him. At the next encounter with my grandparents, they were ready and I led them both in a prayer to accept Jesus Christ as their Savior and Lord.

God generally does not come first to indoctrinate the human mind. He rather pours His love into our hearts.[5] But our minds can be deceived and lofty arguments can bring us to close our heart to God. When we open our hearts to Jesus who brings us to the Father, then we are able to understand and receive the gifts of the Spirit of God.

> "Now we have not received not the spirit of the world, but the Spirit which is from God, that we might understand the gifts bestowed on us by God. And we impart this in words not taught by human wisdom but taught by the Spirit, interpreting spiritual truths to those who possess the Spirit. The unspiritual man does not receive the gifts of the Spirit of God, for they are folly to him, and he is not able to understand them because they are spiritually discerned" 1 Corinthians 2:12-14.

Use the Weapons

So how does one use weapons that are divinely powerful for destroying speculations and lofty arguments raised up against the knowledge of God? What are those powerful weapons that can destroy fortresses? These are spiritual weapons, not of the flesh, that come from the presence and power of the Holy Spirit dwelling in believers. God does not give us a spirit of timidity or fear, but a spirit of power and of love and of self-control. Those who walk not according to the flesh but according to the Spirit are in a position of authority delegated and instituted by God the Father.

The weapons of our warfare most commonly involve words. Just as God spoke to create, we are made in His image to also speak words of command to call down these strongholds. We can use spiritual weapons over our own thoughts, calling down strongholds and everything raised up against the knowledge of God. We can use our authority as believers to bind or reject such thoughts. We can address our own thoughts in areas where we are vulnerable to temptation. We can bind and drive away anger, greed, gossip, lust, bitterness, and unforgiveness. By revelation of the Holy Spirit and the Word of God we can recognize lofty arguments in opposition to the Word of God. We can speak to these mountains commanding them to move in the name of Jesus.

The Word of God is the foremost weapon that is to be spoken into the unseen realms of principalities and powers in the heavenlies. This is God's eternal purpose for the church – to make the manifold wisdom of God known to these principalities and powers. The church can be occupied with many good things; there are needs everywhere, but God's eternal purpose for the church is to speak to the principalities and powers in the heavenly realms.

Most Christians do not know the authority they have as believers. Of those that do, most do not use it. Of those who know and use their authority in Christ, some do not use it wisely. Believers are given authority over self and over thoughts. When you understand the authority you are under and over, just as the Centurion did, you will have increased faith.

Chapter 17

Forgive and Retain Sins

Forgiveness is the fragrance the blossom leaves on the
heel of the boot that crushes it.[1]

The Centurion knew his position of authority: he was under some and set over others. Jesus saw this in him and marveled at his great faith. So our faith will increase by knowing the same as the Centurion, that is, knowing our position of authority. Here we look at another realm of authority given to believers according to the Word of God: we have authority to forgive and retain sins. Knowing and using this authority given us causes increased faith.

The Power of Forgiveness

Jesus said to His disciples, "If you forgive anyone's sins, their sins are forgiven; if you do not forgive them, they are not forgiven" John 20:23. This is a very serious truth with temporal and eternal consequences. There is great power in the word 'forgive.' It is perhaps the most powerful word we can speak. Forgiveness has more power than any other measure of earthly power. It is more powerful than a rocket engine, more powerful than the force of gravity, more powerful than a tornado, more powerful than an earthquake. These earthly powers will pass away, but forgiveness has eternal effects and hence is more powerful. At the time of Jesus' death, after He spoke the words 'forgive them, for they know not what they do,'[2] there was

127

an earthquake causing the ground to shake. Jesus' death for the forgiveness of sins was far more powerful than that earthquake.

Forgiveness has great power both for the present time and for eternity, but most people do not use the word 'forgive'. Most people rather say 'I'm sorry' or 'I apologize'. Being sorrowful or apologetic does not automatically confer forgiveness. These words are not as strong or effective as the word 'forgive.' The great power of forgiveness is given to us by God and is released when words of forgiveness are spoken from the heart.

We must learn how to speak forgiveness. This usually does not occur naturally or instinctively in us. Forgiveness is more than saying "I understand", "it's OK", "I apologize", or "I'm sorry". When reconciling with another, it's essential to say, 'Will you forgive me?' The offended one also should say, 'I forgive you.' Asking for forgiveness and granting forgiveness unleashes heavenly power. A spiritual law comes into force. Just as the law of gravity is in force in the physical realm, forgiveness is a powerful law that moves both heaven and earth. We all need to learn to use our authority to forgive. We should not assume that we understand forgiveness and how to forgive. This is especially so given how powerful forgiveness is.

The Scriptures instructing us about forgiveness say nothing about feelings, understanding, agreement, or belief. A person can say 'I don't like gravity, I don't understand gravity, I don't agree with the law of gravity, and though others believe in gravity, I don't believe in gravity.' When this person jumps off of something, he will fall despite his feelings, understanding, agreement, or belief system. So it is with the law of forgiveness. Forgiveness comes from our heart and will and overrides emotions, understanding, and beliefs. Forgiveness expressed from the heart causes our eyes to open for understanding, releases God's blessings to manage and heal feelings of hurt or anger, and engages God's promise to work all things together for good for those who love Him and are called according to His purpose.[3]

Without Forgiveness

Nowadays it seems people are reluctant to admit wrongdoing. Instead we often hear explanations, denials, and blame shifting. This is really nothing new as such blame shifting occurred when Adam and Eve first sinned. To so deny responsibility and refuse to admit sinful words, actions, and behaviors removes them from the powerful benefits of forgiveness. To speak this way only brings self-deception. It does not usually convince the ones hearing such excuses. "If we say we have no sin, we deceive ourselves, and the truth is not in us" 1 John 1:8.

The consequences of an unwillingness to forgive are equally powerful. There are strong warnings in Jesus' teaching regarding this fact. If anyone will not forgive, this has consequences that are both temporal and eternal, both earthly and heavenly. "For if you forgive men their trespasses, your heavenly Father also will forgive you; but if you do not forgive men their trespasses, neither will your Father forgive your trespasses" Matthew 6:14-15.

If you will not forgive those who sin against you, neither will your Father in heaven forgive your sins. You can have your Pastor pray for you, a great evangelist pray for you, even Jesus himself, but if you will not forgive, those prayers will not benefit. What great power there also is in unforgiveness. God has given authority to us in this matter of forgiveness. We have a choice to wield either force. Mercy triumphs over judgment for those who are merciful.

What is Forgiveness?

Satan also knows of this great power of forgiveness. He knows the consequences of unforgiveness, yielding to himself a degree of power and control. So his agenda is to confuse and distort the meaning and power of forgiveness, knowing that if he can in any way bring a person to refuse to forgive, then the Father in heaven will also not forgive. He attempts to distort and create misunderstanding, hoping to deter one from expressing and receiving forgiveness. The devil's strategy is to tempt us to think wrongly about this powerful tool.

So we should properly understand the authority we are given to forgive. What is forgiveness and what is it not? How can our thinking misguide us as to what true forgiveness is and is not? First, we consider what forgiveness is not.

Anger and Hurt

Maybe you have heard this: "Well, I did forgive, but I need to keep doing it because I keep taking it back," or "It's hard because I still feel hurt by what was said or done." These are responses heard at times when I ask if the one offended has forgiven their offender. We may be tempted to hold a grudge because of feelings of hurt or anger. Such feelings of hurt or anger over what happened can bring a person to conclude that he is not forgiving or that the forgiveness expressed was not real. This confuses unforgiveness with feelings of hurt or anger.

A mother and her young adult daughter came to me from about three hours away seeking counseling and healing. I explained that I am not a trained counselor, but I would be glad to listen and offer prayer and ministry. The young woman was about thirty years old. Her mother explained that her daughter struggles with severe depression and anxiety. These symptoms began about six years earlier after briefly dating a man who in some way violated her. This daughter was reliving the pain and memories of what had happened then. She could not get past this; it seemed to control her daily existence.

I asked her if she had forgiven him. She immediately almost exploded with emotions of hurt and anger, saying "Why should I forgive him after what he did to me. I have been suffering and he is not." I tried to explain what forgiveness is, attempting to convince her not to carry this with her. I explained that the healing of her hurt and anger begins with forgiveness. I encouraged her to use her will override her hurt and anger and to declare forgiveness. Sadly, she would not listen. Instead she interrupted with more of her frequently rehearsed offenses and complaints. Before long she left my office. I wish I could give a good report about her, but I never did hear from her again. She was angry with me because I did not join in her misery and instead encouraged her to forgive. She could not get beyond her emotional pain and chose not to forgive. She was both unforgiving and wounded inwardly. She was controlled by her suffering and would not choose to forgive.

If a person's heart has been wounded, it will stay wounded until God heals it. Forgiveness is the first step in receiving healing.

Feelings of hurt and anger are best attended to by expressing forgiveness from the heart and will. Our feelings do not determine forgiveness. Forgiveness is an agreement to release a person, to decide not to avenge yourself. Just as a mortgage agreement entitles ownership of a home, whether you feel like making the monthly payment or not, forgiveness is an act of the will coming from the heart and is not dependent on feelings. Feelings of hurt or anger are an indication of the need for God's healing touch, not necessarily the need for forgiveness. If you have forgiven someone, they are forgiven. This is true according to the Word of God, "If you forgive anyone's sins, their sins are forgiven" John 20:23. There is nothing said in this verse about feelings of hurt or anger. Forgiveness comes from a person's will which overrides any feelings associated with the offense. The presence of hurt and anger do not automatically indicate unforgiveness. Feeling the pain of what caused the offence can be an indicator of a need for God's healing touch. Such pain can also be an opportunity for the devil to distort forgiveness and equate it with no longer feeling hurt or anger. Forgiveness does not immediately insure that the hurt or anger is gone, but it is a necessary first step in receiving God's healing for the wounds caused by sin.

Though they are connected, forgiveness should not be confused with hurt or anger. When an offence occurs, especially when it is repeated, we may continue to have hurt and anger stirred up. We are instructed to forgive even seventy times seven such offences, that is to say, keep on forgiving indefinitely. This leads us to another misunderstanding of forgiveness. Forgiveness should not be confused with trust.

Trust

Jesus instructed, "Do not give dogs what is holy; and do not throw your pearls before swine, lest they trample them under foot and turn to attack you" Matthew 7:6. Some people are not worthy of trust. Their repeated actions become a warning sign to others to guard your possessions and yourself. Though untrustworthy, these people are to be forgiven. Why would anyone want to hold onto such offences when they can be released by forgiveness?

Jesus defined forgiveness by dying for all people even while we were yet unrepentant sinners; but we know that Jesus trusted no one, for He knew what was in man.[4] Forgiveness does not require restoration of trust in the one who sinned. It is wise to forgive and guard trust simultaneously. However, forgiveness allows the opportunity for the offender to rebuild trust over time and with actions that may eventually restore trust.

Justice

An injustice often tempts to employ the offended one to attempt pay back, to hold a grudge, and to execute punishment. One who forgives chooses not to avenge himself, but this does not leave the offender unpunished. Forgiveness releases a person and choosing not to hold an offense against that person and refusing to avenge yourself. So forgiveness may be confused with justice by wrongly concluding that it removes punishment from a person who deserves it.

A mother brought her thirteen year old son to me seeking advice and ministry. She said her son had been getting A's in all of his classes, but is now flunking all of them instead. She explained that she and her son were currently involved in a court trial involving a man she had dated for about eighteen months. During this time this man was abusing her son sexually. The mother stated that he would be found guilty and maybe spend a year in prison. She said this was unfair and unjust compared with the sufferings and consequences she and her son would face for the rest of their lives.

I explained that God's justice includes the court system but is not limited to it. He will bring justice completely and truthfully. If she and her son try to make him pay, they will instead bring judgment upon themselves. I advised them to leave judgment to God who is much more capable to judge and punish rightly. I was hoping eventually to lead them in a prayer to forgive this man. As I was explaining what forgiveness is and is not, the mother spoke up saying, "I forgive him." Then her son said the same words. There was nothing outwardly special about these words they spoke. There was no particular emotion or struggle. There was no spiritual epiphany or lightning bolt that struck. They simply used their authority to forgive by speaking words of forgiveness.

A few weeks later I saw them and asked how they were doing. The mother stated her son is getting A's in all his classes again. She said they were told that they would need years of counseling for what had occurred. I followed with these people over the next couple years. They continued to do well and never did attend counseling sessions. How great is the power of forgiveness! Their simple words coming from their heart released God's healing and restoration.

Forgiveness means that you will not seek to repay or get revenge, but it does not mean that the person's sinful act will go unpunished. Our God is a gracious God, but He will repay according to true justice. He desires all people to come to repentance and receive forgiveness. A person who refuses to forgive punishes himself. Refusing to forgive is the true injustice as it was in the parable of the king's wicked servant who was forgiven himself but refused to forgive his debtors.[5] The person who forgives allows God to bring healing and true justice. "Beloved, never avenge yourselves, but leave it to the wrath of God; for it is written, 'Vengeance is mine, I will repay, says the Lord'" Romans 12:19. "For the wrongdoer will be paid back for the wrong he has done, and there is no partiality" Colossians 3:25.

What, then, is it to forgive? Forgiveness is an act of a person's heart and will in obedience to the Word of God. Forgiveness releases a person from the injury or consequences caused by their offence. It is to give up a claim for requital. It refuses to seek revenge. Forgiveness gives up a right to hurt someone because you were hurt. Forgiveness is enacted by stating, "I forgive (*insert name*)." This can be simply a statement coming from your heart and will. It can be in a prayer to God. Forgiveness is also enacted by speaking it face to face with an offender who asks for forgiveness. Forgiveness is not granted because a person deserves it, but because we receive forgiveness from God though undeserving ourselves. Forgiveness is often the first step in regaining control of our lives from emotions of hurt and anger. We are authorized to forgive and retain sins.

Retaining Sins

Jesus also said, "whosoever sins you retain, they are retained." What is it to retain sins? There are several ways to understand retaining sins. First, those who do not believe in Jesus will not receive forgiveness of sin or eternal life. So those who reject Jesus have their sins retained and they stand under the wrath of God. "He who believes and is baptized will be saved, but he who does not believe will be condemned" Mark 16:16.

Secondly, those who do not forgive others will have their own sins retained. "If you do not forgive men their trespasses, neither will your Father forgive your trespasses" Matthew 6:15. "And whenever you stand praying, forgive, if you have anything against any one; so that your Father also who is in heaven may forgive you your trespasses" Mark 11:25. To retain sins refers to a refusal to forgive. We should be quick to forgive as the Lord forgave us. To retain sins in this way is destructive, but yet it is in our realm of authority. You can choose unforgiveness, that is, to retain sins. When so choosing, the Father will not forgive you.

Thirdly, to retain sins can also be a discernment of unrepentant sin in others. Jesus had just breathed the Holy Spirit on His disciples as He said these words about forgiving and retaining sins. He was speaking to everyone there. These disciples, who just received the Holy Spirit, were being equipped for the work of the ministry of the gospel. These were soon to be witnesses and leaders in the advancing of the gospel. They were authorized to withhold the pronouncement of God's forgiveness to those who were not contrite and unrepentant, thereby retaining sins. The authority to forgive and retain sins is a function of leadership and spiritual oversight. A Pastor in a church carries more responsibility and authority to pronounce forgiveness of sins to those who confess and are repentant and may retain sins of those unrepentant.

The story of Ananias and Sapphira is such an example which struck fear among the people. Both Ananias and his wife lied to Peter regarding their possessions and offerings. Peter spoke with authority what was therefore required of them. They both died as a result of their sin. Peter, in his authority as a leader in the church, retained the sins of Ananias and Sapphira.[6]

Elymas, the sorcerer, followed Paul and persistently bothered him while Paul proclaimed the Word of God to the Proconsul. Paul grew weary of his interruptions and turned to rebuke him, causing him to go blind.[7] This is another example of the retention of sins.

Paul addressed the Corinthian church regarding a report of immorality where a man was living with his father's wife. He stated that he pronounced judgment in the name of the Lord Jesus on this man. He gave instructions to them: "you are to deliver this man to Satan for the destruction of the flesh, that his spirit may be saved in the day of the Lord Jesus" 1 Corinthians 5:5.

Again, as recorded in 1 Timothy, Paul turned over a couple to Satan in hope that they would repent. "By rejecting conscience, certain persons have made shipwreck of their faith, among them Hymenaeus and Alexander, whom I have delivered to Satan that they may learn not to blaspheme" 1 Timothy 1:19-20. So the Lord "is forbearing toward you, not wishing that any should perish, but that all should reach repentance" 2 Peter 3:9. Those who reject Jesus and who refuse to forgive others will have consequences that hopefully will bring them out of retention of sin and into repentance and forgiveness of sin. The authority to retain sins in this context brings about consequences which will hopefully bring about repentance.

So the authority to forgive and retain sins is given to all people. Anyone can choose to forgive or not forgive because God has given this power and responsibility to each one. Those who believe in Jesus have received and experienced the forgiveness of their sins from God the Father through His Son Jesus Christ. When filled with the Holy Spirit, the authority to forgive and retain sins is amplified for the purposes of advancing the kingdom of God. Furthermore, church leaders have extra authority and position to oversee the ministry of forgiveness and retention of sins in the body of Christ. "Obey your leaders and submit to them; for they are keeping watch over your souls, as men who will have to give account. Let them do this joyfully, and not sadly, for that would be of no advantage to you" Hebrews 13:17.

Chapter 18

People and Possessions

People

All of us are born into and raised under the authority of our parents or other guardians. Each newborn has no authority over others, except in rare circumstances of inherited royalty or other position. Then as we grow in wisdom and stature and favor with God and people, some people are placed in positions of authority over other people. All authority is given by God. There is no authority except what God has ordained. This often includes some degree of oversight and authority over other people. People acquire authority and position most readily because of faithfulness in the little things.

> "He who is faithful in a very little is faithful also in much; and he who is dishonest in a very little is dishonest also in much" Luke 16:10.

> "And he said to him, 'Well done, good servant! Because you have been faithful in a very little, you shall have authority over ten cities'" Luke 19:17.

> "His master said to him, 'Well done, good and faithful servant; you have been faithful over a little, I will set

you over much; enter into the joy of your master'"
Matthew 25:21.

The Centurion had soldiers under him in the chain of command. He had authority to say, 'Come, go, do this or that,' to certain people. He was very aware of his place in the army and functioned effectively within that realm. Jesus called this great faith. So we should understand whose authority we are under and what people we over whom we are set in charge. With this understanding we will have increased faith.

These realms of authority will vary greatly from one person to another and can vary significantly throughout a person's life. Some of the many examples of authority over other people include parents, teachers, coaches, employers, executives, elders, doctors, police, governors, and judges, to name a few. Most of these positions carry a degree of authority as it pertains to a certain part of a person's life and actions. Only a few positions have authority over all aspects of another person's life. An employer has authority over the employee only according the job description and terms of employment. A teacher has a position of authority relative to the order of the classroom and objectives of the course. These positions of authority may have influence in other areas outside of these realms, but do not carry authority over every dimension and decision of those under them. For example, police have authority to enforce the law, but have no say as to what food you will purchase at the grocery store. A teacher has no authority to run a student's business or financial affairs. A medical doctor can place a person on a 72 hour hold if he is a danger to himself or others, but this doctor otherwise only makes recommendations and offers treatments.

Parents and Children

There are some positions of authority that are all encompassing. Most common is the position of a father and mother who watch over and are responsible for all matters involving their child or children. "Children, obey your parents *in everything*, for this pleases the Lord.

Fathers, do not provoke your children, lest they become discouraged"
Colossians 3. 20-21 (Italics mine).

Children are instructed to obey their parents in everything
because parents have authority over every aspect of their child's life.
When parents send a child to school, they are delegating some of the
responsibility and authority to the teachers, but still retain the overall
duty to train up their child in the way he should go. The authority of
parents over their children involves every aspect of their lives. As
children grow and become more responsible and trustworthy, they
should be given responsibility and decision making powers according
to their age, development, and ability. However the overall authority
yet rests with the parents. Parents have the duty to instruct their child
to understand and obey them. This is an essential lesson for their
safety, blessings, and well-being. Failure to establish this obedience
to parental authority essentially means that the child at least thinks
he or she determines the course of things at home or may be actually
running the household at times.

We have all seen a mother or father with their child at the grocery
store or some other shopping venue, saying 'no' at first in a normal
voice. Then as the child continues the undesired behavior, 'no' is said
again, maybe with a little more sternness. Yet the behavior continues
and 'no' is repeated several times louder and louder until everyone
around can hear mom or dad shouting. Every parent has encountered
something like this when raising their own children. We can be inad-
vertently teaching the child that 'no' does not mean 'no' until it is
spoken several times with increasing volume and eventually anger.

Teaching a child the importance of obedience and the word 'no' is
not an easy task, but failure to establish obedience at home spills over
to disobedience to other authorities including God Himself. Teaching
and expecting obedience from children imparts faith. The Centurion
possessed, comprehended, and operated under and in this obedience
that Jesus called faith. Jesus himself learned obedience.[1]

The blessings and benefits of obedience to authority at home
fulfil a commandment and engage a promise from God: so that it
may go well with you and that you will enjoy long life on earth. All
of us should honor our father and mother, no matter how old you
or they are. All parents are sinners, none are perfect. Yet we are to

honor them regardless, so that life would go well for us and that we would enjoy long life on the earth. Children are to obey their parents in the Lord. Fathers are to raise up children in the training and instruction of the Lord, and not cause them to stumble or disobey our heavenly Father.

> "Children, obey your parents in the Lord, for this is right. 'Honor your father and mother'—which is the first commandment with a promise— 'so that it may go well with you and that you may enjoy long life on the earth.' Fathers, do not exasperate your children; instead, bring them up in the training and instruction of the Lord" Ephesians 6:1-4.

As previously established, authority exists for blessing, protection, and provision. Every parent has this position and duty and authority to provide, bless, and protect.

Husbands and Wives

Another common all-encompassing position of authority is the role of a husband who watches over his wife. This concept is not popular in today's culture. Nevertheless, it is soundly biblical throughout all Scriptures. We should have a biblical view of our culture, rather than a cultural interpretation of the Bible. Did I already state that authority exists for purposes of blessing, protection, and provision? God set up His created order to give extra honor and protection to wives under the authority of their husbands. A husband has a special place before God to love his wife, pray for her, honor and keep her.

> "Wives, be subject to your husbands, as is fitting in the Lord" Colossians 3:18.

> "Likewise you wives, be submissive to your husbands, so that some, though they do not obey the word, may be won without a word by the behavior of their wives, when they see your reverent and chaste behavior. Let

not yours be the outward adorning with braiding of hair, decoration of gold, and wearing of fine clothing, but let it be the hidden person of the heart with the imperishable jewel of a gentle and quiet spirit, which in God's sight is very precious. So once the holy women who hoped in God used to adorn themselves and were submissive to their husbands, as Sarah obeyed Abraham, calling him lord. And you are now her children if you do right and let nothing terrify you. Likewise you husbands, live considerately with your wives, bestowing honor on the woman as the weaker sex, since you are joint heirs of the grace of life, in order that your prayers may not be hindered" 1 Peter 3:1-7.

This role of authority and subjection between husbands and wives reflects the very nature of God. This kind of relationship is the essence of the Trinity, where the Son and the Holy Spirit are subject to the Father in everything. The Word of God also uses this relationship to describe Christ and the church.

"Be subject to one another out of reverence for Christ. Wives, be subject to your husbands, as to the Lord. For the husband is the head of the wife as Christ is the head of the church, his body, and is himself its Savior. As the church is subject to Christ, so let wives also be subject *in everything* to their husbands. Husbands, love your wives, as Christ loved the church and gave himself up for her, that he might sanctify her, having cleansed her by the washing of water with the word, that he might present the church to himself in splendor, without spot or wrinkle or any such thing, that she might be holy and without blemish. Even so husbands should love their wives as their own bodies. He who loves his wife loves himself" Ephesians 5.21-28 (Italics mine).

Consider Your Position

As an exercise in acquiring increased faith, we should all carefully consider our position in life. Like a brick in a wall that has some bricks above it, some below, and some alongside, we have people above, below, and alongside us. We are to submit to the 'bricks' set over us as they are God's delegated authorities for our blessing, protection, and provision. Those 'bricks' we are set over are ones that benefit from the oversight, example, prayers, and provision we can provide. The bricks alongside each other are other people where there is no direct relationship of authority. These are people under someone else's authority, perhaps the same authority you may also be under, like the relationship of a co-worker. These people are under God's authority whether submitting to Him or not and they benefit from our prayers.

Each of us should examine our situation in life and recognize those in authority over us and the extent of authority we might have over others. We have established that a biblical definition of faith includes authority, understanding and using it wisely. Paul's instructions in Romans 12 call us to do this very thing. We are to think of ourselves appropriately according to the amount of authority (faith) God has given.[2] God assigns to each of us a measure of faith which is a measure of authority. We should assess our position, like bricks in a wall, to understand with sober judgment the authority we have been given, being careful not to think you are a different brick in a higher (or lower) position.

Since all authority comes from God and there is no authority except what is instituted by God, anyone in any position of authority is to represent God and serve His purposes. So there are clear instructions in Scripture for those in positions of authority over others.

"But Jesus called them to him and said, "You know that the rulers of the Gentiles lord it over them, and their great men exercise authority over them. It shall not be so among you; but whoever would be great among you must be your servant, and whoever would be first among you must be your slave; even as the Son

of man came not to be served but to serve, and to give
His life as a ransom for many" Matthew 20:25-28.

"Masters, treat your slaves justly and fairly, knowing
that you also have a Master in heaven" Colossians 4:1.

"So I exhort the elders among you, as a fellow elder
and a witness of the sufferings of Christ as well as a
partaker in the glory that is to be revealed. Tend the
flock of God that is your charge, not by constraint
but willingly, not for shameful gain but eagerly, not
as domineering over those in your charge but being
examples to the flock. And when the chief Shepherd
is manifested you will obtain the unfading crown of
glory. Likewise you that are younger be subject to
the elders. Cloth yourselves, all of you, with humility
toward one another, for "God opposes the proud, but
gives grace to the humble" 1 Peter 5:1-5.

Possessions

You are the one who is responsible for what you own. You are able
to make choices about your possessions because you have authority
to do so by virtue of ownership. God is most interested in speaking
to you about the things He has entrusted to you since you are directly
in charge. You may consult an auto mechanic for advice about your
car, but what happens to your car is your decision. Your computer
may malfunction causing you to seek advice and repair, but this is
your choice as the owner.

One cold January day, -30 degrees Fahrenheit, I awoke on a Sunday
morning to get ready for church. When I turned on the hot water, there
was nothing that came out of the faucet. I knew the pipe was frozen
with the extreme cold weather. I also knew that in a short time the pipe
could not withstand the expanding frozen water and would burst. I was
perplexed because the water pipe supplying hot water to the bathtub
was not located along an outside wall of the house where it would be
exposed to freezing temperatures. Also it was the hot water supply that

was frozen. The cold water was running. I knelt with my wife in prayer in my bedroom and asked God to guide me to where the frozen pipe was located. I did not want to or have time to tear out the whole wall looking for the problem. I was mindful that it was my responsibility as I was the owner of this home. No one else would jump in to take responsibility for this matter. I prayed with faith as a result of understanding the authority God has given over one's possessions.

I knew the builder of the home and gave him a phone call. He was also perplexed why this pipe would freeze. He called me back a few minutes later with information that he felt would identify where the frozen pipe was located. He took me around the corner into the laundry room and described to me over the phone where I should place my drill to cut into the wall board. I looked at a wall with no particular markings. I pointed the drill at the exact spot to describe to me over the phone and began to drill through the drywall. The drill bit did not punch through the drywall, but hit the copper pipe precisely where it was frozen. I cut out a small part of the drywall and used the heat from a hairdryer to thaw the frozen pipe before it ruptured.

I was thankful that I did not have water damage to my home, but I was also struck with the understanding of what had just happened. My position of ownership and associated authority over my home brought my wife and me to a place of prayer with faith and authority. The Lord provided an answer to prayer through the builder.

We have authority over the items we own. So we can make decisions about our possessions. God provides abundantly for the things we need such as food, clothing, and shelter. We are instructed not to worry about these things because our Father in heaven knows you need them, but all the other stuff we accumulate can begin to rule our lives. Our possessions are to be under our authority. When we lay up treasure in things we can eventually become a slave to those things. Lay up treasure in heaven where moth and rust cannot consume.

> "And he said to them, 'Take heed, and beware of all covetousness; for a man's life does not consist in the abundance of his possessions. And he told them a parable, saying, 'The land of a rich man brought forth plentifully; and he thought to himself, "What shall

I do, for I have nowhere to store my crops?" And he said, "I will do this: I will pull down my barns, and build larger ones; and there I will store all my grain and my goods. And I will say to my soul, Soul, you have ample goods laid up for many years; take your ease, eat, drink, be merry." But God said to him, "Fool! This night your soul is required of you; and the things you have prepared, whose will they be?" So is he who lays up treasure for himself, and is not rich toward God.' ... For where your treasure is, there will your heart be also" Luke 12:15-21, 34.

It was a great blessing for me to visit Christians in Russia soon after the wall of the cold war came down. I met many believers and heard their stories of faith, including the testimonies of some of the old-timers who spoke of spending twenty years in prison because of their faith in Jesus Christ. They counted it a great privilege to serve the Lord in prison rather than deny their faith in Jesus. I spoke with one of these men after a church service. He said, "Where are you from?" I stated I was from the USA. He said, "It must be so difficult for you there." I was wondering if I heard the interpreter correctly and asked him to repeat. He said again, "It must be so difficult there for Christians in your country because you have so much." These Russian Christians did not grow up in the affluence of my culture. They had spent years in prison for their faith, yet considered it more difficult for me to live as a Christian in my culture. It is a challenge to manage the great accumulation of stuff we have while continuing to walk in the Spirit.

With ownership comes responsibility. Every possession can demand time and more money. This time and money can be given to the Lord and others. It is God's pleasure to provide what we need. The more we own the more resources of our time, energy, and money is required. It can seem that our possessions can thus have authority over us and this ought not to be so.

Each one has authority over their possessions. Some people have authority over other people. An understanding of position in life and the authority a believer has, involves consideration of what people and possessions over which God has placed us.

Chapter 19

Diseases and Infirmities

———————✦———————

Healing occurs in a variety of ways. Healing or resolution of symptoms can occur by natural means, lifestyle changes, medical therapy, and by supernatural intervention.

Natural Healing

Our bodies have amazing normal repair processes. This natural healing is from God who created us with these characteristics. When skin is lacerated, a natural built in process of healing begins. When blood vessels are ruptured, the muscle fibers in the wall of vessel near the injury constrict to lessen the amount of blood loss. Blood flow out from a wound helps cleanse the injured area. A clot forms when blood stops flowing from the wound to assist in wound repair. (Blood has an incredible ability to remain as a liquid when flowing and thicken or clot when not flowing.) When an ankle is sprained, chemical signals called cytokines are released. These cytokines contribute to increased blood flow to the injured area bringing macrophages, white blood cells, nutrients, and other sources for repair. This causes some swelling and is a natural bodily response to injury. These are just a few, among very many, examples of natural healing. God made us with certain innate and automatic tools to repair and rebuild injured or diseased areas in our bodies.

Lifestyle Changes

Lifestyle changes can sometimes bring our bodies back to more normal functions. Sometimes our bodies are speaking to us with symptoms that may indicate a need for change. Feeling tired can indicate a need for sleep or a need for exercise or improved diet. If you touch your hand on a burner, a very quick reaction occurs to protect from injury. Some musculoskeletal symptoms are evidence of an overuse injury. If a person suddenly cannot hear well from one ear, it could be plugged with cerumen. There are many such symptoms that give us messages, some obvious and others not so clear. We do not get a text message or email from our body; instead we get symptoms that sometimes communicate a need for change or corrective cares.

Again, as with natural healing, this is how God created us. Our bodies give us feedback so we learn to care for ourselves and make appropriate adjustments. Seeking supernatural healing for such symptoms without understanding and heeding these bodily messages seeks to bypass or disregard the care we owe to the members of our being. An ear plugged with cerumen needs to be cleaned. This is not a matter requiring supernatural intervention. If your hand is on a hot object, you will take it away to avoid any further injury because you understand clearly the message your nerves are sending to your brain. No one would keep a hand on a hot burner in order to pause and pray for the pain and burning to stop.

A crowd had been with Jesus all day as He taught them and healed the sick. The disciples asked Jesus if they should send them home to get something to eat as they were in a lonely place. Some of them may have become lightheaded without sufficient food and water. There is no record of Jesus healing the symptom of lightheadedness among these people; rather He fed the crowd. Those who may have felt symptoms from lack of food and water did not receive healing of those symptoms. Rather Jesus attended to what their symptoms pointed to – He fed them.[1]

Medical Therapy

Most medicines function to assist the body in doing its regular functions. One could argue that this is not actual healing, but instead medicines are helping the body to function better in an ongoing disease state. Jesus did not oppose the healing remedies of His day. Sometimes He used them as means for spiritual or supernatural healing. When Jesus spit on the ground to mix it with dirt and applied this to the eyes of a blind man, some report that He was using a remedy of that time period along with His supernatural healing power.

As you might expect, I do not see a conflict between God's divine healing and most medicines. My strategy is to seek first the kingdom of God and His righteousness. Consider what the symptoms may be suggesting in regard to a change of activity. Use the authority as a believer to address the disease or infirmity. If there is no change in symptoms, be free to use over-the-counter medications as directed and seek advice and treatment from a doctor if needed.

Supernatural Healing

God brings healing through natural and medical methods. He also heals supernaturally, that is, by divine intervention apart from or in addition to natural means. This can be an increased rate of the normal natural healing process. It can be a change of anatomy and symptoms by God's healing power. Supernatural healing can occur instantly or over some hours, days, or weeks. These serve to demonstrate the presence of the kingdom of God and bring confirmation to the Word of God. They function as signs of the compassion and majesty of God.

There are 41 stories recorded in the four gospels about Jesus or His disciples ministering healing to others. The number of verses describing these events, and associated instructions about healing, occupy almost 20% of all the verses in the Gospels of Matthew, Mark, Luke, and John. There are 3779 verses in these four gospels. 727 of them have to do with healing of physical and mental problems and discussions about these events. Moral healing is much less discussed.

Numerous stories of healing are also documented in other New and Old Testament Scriptures.

Despite this prominence of discussion about physical healing in the Bible, so many Christian believers and churches are uninformed as to how to bring divine healing to others. Some struggle to believe that God heals today. Preaching about these biblical stories many times gets spiritualized. For example, when Jesus healed the blind men they obviously received the physical ability to see, but some preaching today focuses on spiritual blindness. When the ten lepers were cleansed, the message might be about the one who returned to give thanks to Jesus. Though these are worthwhile scriptural lessons, the main point of these accounts is to demonstrate the presence of the kingdom of God by illustrating God's healing of the physical body through Jesus and His disciples.

Most church leaders and attenders today do not recognize Jesus' emphasis on the works of the kingdom of God. They have been spiritualized or overlooked, while the focus instead is on teaching doctrine and moral living. By and large the church today has not understood healing and often questions if God wants to heal. We do not usually question if God wants to forgive, but we do routinely question if God wants to heal.

Sometimes sickness is described as God's will for those who suffer. These same people would never send their children to a teacher who inflicted illness upon the students so that they would learn lessons. God is sometimes viewed in this way, allowing or even causing illness in order that we may learn lessons. Certainly God uses trials including diseases to bring us to Him and we can learn and grow from them. He promises to work all things, including diseases and infirmities, together for good for those who love Him. But if someone believes it is not God's will to heal, then going to a doctor for help would be opposing God's will.

Sin and Sickness

There is a connection between diseases and sins. Some diseases and injuries are the direct consequence of sin. Seeking forgiveness from God brings cleansing by the shed blood of Jesus and may undo some or all of these consequences. Diseases and infirmities came to this world as a result of the fall of mankind into sin, but we should not conclude that every disease is directly related to some specific sin. It is not a sin to be sick or injured.

> "And behold, they brought to him a paralytic, lying on his bed; and when Jesus saw their faith he said to the paralytic, 'Take heart, my son, your sins are forgiven.' And behold, some of the scribes said to themselves, 'This man is blaspheming.' But Jesus, knowing their thoughts, said, 'Why do you think evil in your hearts? For which is easier to say, "Your sins are forgiven"; or to say, "Rise and walk"? But that you might know that the Son of man has authority on earth to forgive sins' – he then said to the paralytic – 'Rise, take up your bed and go home.' And he rose and went home. When the crowds saw it, they were afraid, and they glorified God, who had given such authority to men" Matthew 9:1-8.

When Jesus healed this paralytic, Jesus used the occasion to demonstrate His authority to forgive by healing the paralytic. The visible healing of paralysis occurred by the same word of Jesus to pronounce forgiveness, which is not so visible. Jesus had asked the Pharisees, "which is easier to say, 'Your sins are forgiven' or 'Rise, take up your bed and walk?' The Pharisees could say neither one. Both of these statements could not come from their mouths.

For Christians today, it is much easier to say 'your sins are forgiven' than to say 'rise, take up your bed, and walk.' It is easier to state something that is not so measurable than to tell someone to do something they cannot do except by a miracle of God. Both forgiveness and physical healing are miraculous provisions from God, but our faith in the forgiveness of sins exceeds our faith in instant divine healing.

Jesus could say both statements as He knew His authority to forgive and to heal. He demonstrated forgiveness and healing, and then He instructed His disciples to do the same as He gave them this authority to forgive and heal. They were able to say both, 'Your sins are forgiven', and 'Rise, take up your bed and go home.' The obvious scriptural answer regarding God's will to forgive and heal is 'yes' to both.

Jesus asked another question of the Pharisees: "Why do you think evil in your hearts?" The Pharisees were questioning and opposing Jesus' authority to forgive sins. Jesus called this evil thinking. It is evil to oppose God's works of forgiveness and healing. It is evil because these leaders of the synagogue were using their positions of authority to withhold God's grace of forgiveness and healing from coming to the people. It is evil because God's forgiveness and healing comes from His holy nature. God yearns to attend to the people He loves greatly.

We see this nature of God to heal in His Son Jesus who said to the Centurion, "I will come and heal him." Jesus did not stop to look at His calendar and schedule an appointment. He did not inquire about the nature of the servant's physical condition. He did not ask if the servant believed in him or if he believed in God's power to heal. He did not check into the moral worthiness of this servant or the Centurion. He did not focus on his sins or shortcomings. Jesus spontaneously responded from the heart of His Father to offer to heal the servant immediately. Jesus, who does nothing of His own will, but only what He sees the Father doing, said, "I will come and heal him." Matthew 8:7. This displayed the nature of the Father whose very name is Jehovah Raphah, the Lord your healer.

Authority to Heal

So what authority regarding healing is given to the believer? Matthew 10:1 says: "And he called to him His twelve disciples and gave them authority over unclean spirits, to cast them out, and to heal every disease and every infirmity." This authority was given to His twelve disciples. Did Jesus intend this authority given to these twelve would stop with them or does it extend beyond them to other believers?

There are accounts of healing in the New and Old Testaments performed by others than these twelve. Most notable in the New

Testament is the Apostle Paul. There are numerous records of healing by Paul's ministry. Paul demonstated and taught about the gifts of the Spirit including healing. His writings to the Corinthians state that the gifts of the Holy Spirit are given to each one as the Spirit wills. All of these gifts, services, and workings are inspired in everyone. So the gifts of healing are inspired by the Holy Spirit in all believers.

> "Now there are varieties of gifts, but the same Spirit; and there are varieties of service, but the same Lord; and there are varieties of working, but it is the same God who *inspires them all in every one. To each* is given the manifestation of the Spirit for the common good" 1 Corinthians 12:4-7 (Italics mine).

Additionally, we can see from the great commission that Jesus intended this authority to be given to all believers. Jesus taught His disciples about how to bring healing to others in His name. He said, "Heal the sick, raise the dead, cleanse lepers, cast out demons. You have received without paying, give without pay" Matthew 10:8. Later in the great commission, He instructed these same disciples to make disciples of all nations, teaching them to obey everything He had commanded them. What had He commanded them? Jesus had commanded His disciples to heal the sick, raise the dead, cleanse lepers, and cast out demons. Now these disciples were to teach others to obey what He had commanded them: heal the sick, raise the dead, cleanse lepers, and cast out demons. The authority to heal every disease and every infirmity is thereby given to every believer. This extends the authority to heal to all believers in all nations.

This authority is to be taught to new disciples according to the great commission. Healing does not usually automatically happen among new disciples. It needs to be taught, just as Jesus instructed and authorized His disciples. Though sometimes God heals sovereignly, He prefers to use His people to bring His healing to others. God has prioritized the release of His healing power to flow through believers and thereby restricted Himself through His people. This is why Jesus challenged His disciples for their lack of faith.[2] It was better for Jesus to go to the Father so the Holy Spirit would come alongside believers to continue His ministry.

> "And Jesus came and said to them, 'All authority in heaven and on earth has been given to me. Go therefore and make disciples of all nations, baptizing them in the name of the Father and of the Son and of the Holy Spirit, *teaching them to observe all that I have commanded you*, and lo, I am with you always, to the close of the age'" Matthew 28:18-20 (Italics mine).

Every Disease and Every Infirmity

The authority given to believers is over every disease and every infirmity. There is no disease or weakness that is excluded. All manner of conditions are included in the authority to heal that Jesus gives to His disciples. There are no exceptions here. There are no diseases or weaknesses that fall outside of this authority Jesus gives to His disciples. This authority was given regardless of how much is known about diseases and their pathological mechanisms. It is not necessary to become a doctor to bring healing to others. Medical knowledge is not required. It is not even necessary to know the name of the disease or infirmity.

Jesus did say to the apostles' request for increased faith, "You shall say to THIS mountain, move from here to there and it will obey you." This was not speaking to any mountain. THIS mountain is a specific mountain, a specific disease or illness with a specific pathologic mechanism. Most diseases have many related symptoms and can involve many organs in the human body. Yet most diseases can be explained by a single underlying pathology causing certain symptoms.

When I attended medical school, I was especially tuned into these mechanisms of disease. I wanted insight into how to direct a word of command to THIS mountain. I was interested in learning how and where to release the resurrection power present in a believer to minister healing to others. Jesus' words, "Move from here to there," also had some specificity. It was not simply addressing the mountain by name.

The command had a 'here' and a 'there.' Where is 'here' and 'there' when ministering healing? What needs to move for each disease? I wanted to understand how to issue a word of command to the underlying physical cause for each disease and its associated symptoms.

Just as an electrician has understanding about an electrical circuit and can identify the cause of a malfunction, so it is possible for believers to identify THIS mountain and speak a word of command to a specific matter telling it to move or do something. Just as an electrician never doubts the presence and power of electricity when troubleshooting a circuit, so a believer should never doubt the will and power of God to heal, but consider how to address the crux of the problem. When we do not see healing happen, we have questioned God's will and power rather than the circuit through which His power flows.

The pathological basis of diseases varies with each disease, but many diseases can be categorized according to similar mechanisms for the purposes of considering how to speak to 'this mountain.' In the next chapters I have categorized some common diseases according to similar mechanisms of pathology. This is by no means a complete rendition of every disease and every infirmity by today's knowledge of physiology and pathology. It is a simplified, condensed review of some of the basics with the hope that this will be helpful when considering how to use the authority of a Spirit-filled believer to speak to the mountain of a disease.

The following chapters include discussion about diseases grouped in these categories: autoimmune diseases, mutations, infections, infirmities and injuries, endocrine, and behavioral diseases. Discussions about these conditions include the underlying mechanism of disease along with instructions and strategies for specifically speaking a word of command to these various diseases and infirmities. We are given authority over every disease and every infirmity. Let's consider then how to use this authority to speak to each disease and infirmity in the name of Jesus Christ. Let's understand some of the nature of these diseases so we can address what needs to move from here to there. Jesus said, "If you have faith, you will say to this mountain, 'move from here to there', and it will obey you" Matthew 17:20. Let's look at where here and there might be for diseases in each of these categories.

Section 3

MECHANISMS OF DISEASE

In the first section we have established an understanding of faith. Faith submits to those in authority over us and faith knows what position of authority we have been given. The second section outlines these realms of authority in detail.

This third section further unpacks the believer's authority over every disease and every infirmity by categorizing common diseases according to similar mechanisms of pathology. This is an oversimplified look at the causes of diseases in order to gain insight as to where to direct God's power by word of command. For each disease state, what is the specific mountain that can be spoken to? What it is that needs to move from here to there? Where is here and where is there when speaking authoritatively to diseases and infirmities?

The following is not an exhaustive list of diseases and infirmities; rather it is a review of some common mechanisms of disease.

Chapter 20

Autoimmune Diseases

Immunity

The immune system provides a remarkably effective defense system that ensures that, although we spend our lives surrounded by potentially pathogenic microorganisms, we become ill only relatively rarely, and when infection occurs it is usually met successfully and is followed by lasting immunity.

The immune system is a truly incredible and amazing function of the human body. The various components and functions that comprise the immune system include white blood cells, T cells, B helper cells, the lymphatic system, the thymus gland, and the spleen. Together these parts of the immune system distinguish self from non-self. These are constantly scanning and looking for epitopes that signal to the immune system that something foreign is present. Epitopes are molecules on the surface of organisms or foreign objects that the immune system recognizes as non-self. When recognizing something as not self, various components of the immune system will attack and remove, if possible, what is invading.

The immune system acquires a sense of self, enabling it to distinguish self when compared to another organism or foreign object. Even identical twins have immune systems that distinguish one from another. A kidney can be transplanted from one human to another but the immune system will recognize this transplanted kidney as not self. This is why antirejection drugs are required when a transplant of one human organ to another person occurs. This graft rejection is less aggressive in family members and others who have similar molecular identities.

This one unique feature of every human being, among many countless other amazing facts of human anatomy, points to how we are truly fearfully and wonderfully made. The amazing immune system shouts out loudly and clearly to disprove the theory of evolution. How could it be that each one would accidentally acquire his own amazing clarity of identity and protection against disease? It can only be at the hands of our loving Creator.

A pregnant mother who has Rh negative blood type has an immune system that will attack her baby if she encounters some of a baby's Rh positive blood. So a medicine called Rhogam is given to the mother to prevent this process of rejection in the event of a miscarriage or other bleeding. A woman should have control over her own body, but a baby in her womb is not her own body. This is a different body with a different blood type.

As a baby forms in the womb, its DNA genetic code is unique. In the process of fetal development, a human being acquires identity. The immune system begins to recognize this sense of self early on. At birth each one of us is exposed to an external environment. At this time our immune system is rather naïve and begins to sort out self from the surrounding environment. Sometimes a newborn child will exhibit various benign rashes on the skin that are representative of his or her immune system which is learning self from nonself. During this time and up to five or six months after birth an infant benefits from passive immunity coming from the mother through the placenta before birth. Passive immunity is the mother's immune memory and response to the diseases she has encountered passed on to her child first through the placenta, then after delivery through breast milk.

During childhood years frequent infections and illnesses occur. Childhood cough and cold symptoms are most commonly caused by viruses. Parents and grandparents of these children may not get the same infection because they have usually been exposed to the particular virus or something similar. Their immune system is ready to fight it off before an infection occurs. As the immune system continues to learn and acquire memory of various pathogens, a more rapid response is mounted to prevent systemic symptoms.

Vaccinations are given to train the immune system to fight against disease without actually being exposed to the disease itself. This training of the immune system is a process of acquiring a quick response to battle against infection. Though we do not have vaccinations for every infection, the vaccinations we do have are usually very effective. They have almost eradicated certain diseases. Consequently, we have almost forgotten how devastating and serious were such diseases as polio, measles, smallpox, mumps, etc. Many people do remember chickenpox for which we now have a vaccination. Prior to this vaccination there was an intentional effort to expose children to chickenpox to prevent more virulent symptoms and possible complication during pregnancy. Before the varicella vaccination about 100 infants died each year from chickenpox. I want to simply underscore how important it is to receive vaccinations and stay current on them.

The immune system is comprised of the histamine system, B cells and T cells, the lymphatic system and lymph nodes, the spleen, and other types of cells that are circulating in the blood such as mast cells and eosinophils. They each have specific functions and work together to preserve health and fight off disease. This is God's gift of health to us built into our anatomy.

Errors of Immunity

There are errors that can occur causing certain diseases we call autoimmune diseases. These are diseases where the immune system mistakenly attacks self instead of non-self. Sometimes an epitope is perceived to be foreign when in fact it is not.

There are many types of autoimmune diseases but all of them have in common this one feature: the immune system attacking self. Rheumatoid arthritis, for example, occurs when the immune system attacks joints and the fluid in the joints. Diabetes mellitus, type I, is where the immune system errantly attacks the beta islet cells in the pancreas so that they no longer can produce insulin. (Diabetes mellitus, type II, is not an autoimmune disease but is a result of increased insulin resistance due to various factors discussed in chapter about endocrine diseases.) Autoimmune hemolytic anemia occurs when the spleen attacks and chews up red blood cells. Other autoimmune diseases include Psoriasis, Scleroderma, Myasthenia Gravis, Multiple Sclerosis, Guillian Barre, Sjogren's Disease, Psoriatic Arthritis, Dermatomyositis, Lupus, Reynauds, Autoimmune Hemolytic Anemia, Sjogren's disease, Autoimmune Thyroid Disease (Hashimoto or Graves), Celiac Disease, Hypoparathyroidism, Primary Ovarian Insufficiency, Primary Gonadal (testes) Failure, and Pernicious Anemia.

Allergy and Hypersensitivity

Sometimes parts of the immune system overreact to various antigens causing allergy symptoms. This is really not an autoimmune disease because it is the immune system attacking non-self, but the attack against these antigens is excessive. An allergy reaction is a hypersensitivity reaction.

Allergic reactions occur when an individual, who has produced an antibody in response to an innocuous antigen or allergen, subsequently encounters the same antigen. This triggers the activation of IgE-binding mast cells in the exposed tissue, leading to a series of responses that are characteristic of allergy. Though rarely life-threatening, it causes much distress and lost time from work and school. Our immune system can learn to coexist with a certain amount of repeated exposures to these antigens to eventually diminish allergy symptoms.

There are circumstances when this allergy mechanism is protective, especially in response to parasitic worms, which are prevalent in underdeveloped countries. In more advanced countries, however, where there is not much problem with worms, IgE immune responses to innocuous antigens predominate, and allergy is one of the most prevalent diseases. Allergy symptoms affect up to half of the populations of developed countries.

A member of my church was a missionary in Ecuador for four years. He heard me describe this relationship between hypersensitivity reactions in more developed countries and worms are parasites in less developed countries. He confirmed this to be true for him.

While residing in the USA, he had frequent allergy symptoms. While in Ecuador, he had no allergy symptoms, but had to be routinely treated for worms and parasites. I have participated in twenty short term missions for purposes of evangelism, teaching, construction, and medical care. I do not remember ever encountering or treating anyone with asthma on any of these mission trips. Frequently there were encounters with people infested with worms and parasites.

Asthma is always related to certain triggers, some of which are extrinsic (allergens) and others are intrinsic (internal conditions or exercise induced). The disease Asthma can be understood in part by its hypersensitivity reaction to these triggers.

How to Minister

Though it is not necessary to understand these mechanisms of diseases for ministering God's healing power, I am giving you some basic insight into the disease processes so that you can be more specific in speaking to 'this mountain'. For autoimmune diseases it is appropriate to address the immune system, instructing it in the name of Jesus to stop attacking self. For example, when ministering to a person with autoimmune hemolytic anemia, we can speak to the spleen and command it to stop sequestering and removing normal healthy blood cells. For someone with rheumatoid arthritis we can speak to the immune system to stop attacking the joints. You can also address the pain, stiffness, swelling and deformity that may result from the misguided activity of the immune system. For someone with allergy symptoms, we can speak to the histamine system, mast cells, and eosinophils to stop overreacting to harmless allergens. For those with asthma, speak to the bronchiole and alveoli spasms telling them to relax and command the mucus production to dissipate.

Physical healing from God occurs by faith in the name of Jesus Christ who lives and dwells in believers through the Holy Spirit. When we learn to release that power within us, through the laying on of hands and word of command, healings occur. It is not required or mandatory to know any medical facts or the mechanisms of anatomy and physiology for a believer to be a vessel through which divine healing flows. Jesus said that we will speak to 'this mountain' and it will obey us when we have a small amount of faith like a grain of mustard seed. This is not mustered up faith; it is mustard seed faith. 'YOU SHALL SAY' to 'this mountain' simply speaks to the basic mechanism causing disease, telling it to move from 'here' to 'there.' The primary cause of immune system related disorders is a misguided immunity that either attacks self or is overreacting.

Chapter 21

Mutations

Perhaps no one word, describing all the diseases we know about, strikes more fear than the word 'cancer.' Everyone knows someone afflicted with some type of cancer and everyone knows of someone who has died as a result of this type of disease. Some types of cancers are very virulent and others are more indolent. Pancreatic cancer is very difficult to detect in its early stages and has a high morbidity and mortality rate. Conversely, prostate cancer in men is something most men will get eventually and die with it rather than die from it. (Some prostate cancers are aggressive and do cause early morbidity and mortality.)

There are over 200 different types of cancers, but they all have three characteristics in common. It's helpful to understand these characteristics for guidance as to how to speak to "this mountain." Additionally, there are parallels with our spiritual lives when we understand the mechanisms of cancer.

Just what is cancer? There are many different types of cancer. There are cancers of the blood, sarcomas, adenomas, carcinomas, soft tissue cancers, and cancers that originate from almost every organ in the body. Each cancer has its own features and complications that can occur when certain cells of an organ in the body mutate and transform into something else. These mutations can occur from injury to the DNA or from errors in DNA replication when cells divide.

DNA is a double helical strand. You've probably seen pictures of what DNA might look like. During cell division the two strands of DNA unwind and unzip. Then different types of RNA create a complementary strand to each of the unzipped strands. Another type of RNA then looks over and proofreads the new DNA strands for errors. This whole process of cell division is amazingly accurate with an error rate of 1 in 1,000,000 to 1 in 10,000,000 pairings. But errors do occur which over time can result in a cell that becomes cancerous. This cell can sometimes replicate itself reproducing these errors.

Cancer Characteristics

Every type of cancer has 3 basic characteristics: 1) cancer cells lose their identity and function; 2) cancer cells do not die when they are supposed to; and 3) cancer cells are able to spread to other organs and areas of the body.[1]

Loss of Identity and Function.

I had the opportunity and privilege to attend 29 years of school. The two classes that were the most worshipful for me were astronomy and embryology. In my astronomy class my mind was stretched to its limit trying to comprehend the vastness of creation. In my embryology class we learned the amazing and miraculous formation of a human being from an egg and sperm which contain a unique DNA genetic code.

This genetic code present in every living cell in the human body contains all the information to code for the formation and function of every organ in the body. As the fertilized egg divides and forms the morula and blastula, these cells initially form an outer layer (ectoderm), a middle layer (mesoderm), and inner layer (endoderm). Then these cells each later take on more specific identities and functions as they become various organs. This occurs as the DNA coding for forming a specific organ switches off the other information in the DNA that codes for all the other organs. So as the liver is being formed, those cells somehow know their identity and together they become a liver. So this liver will not contain lung cells or kidney cells.

Though the liver cells contain all the information in the genetic code of DNA, only the specific codings for the liver are turned on to produce cells that look like and function like a liver. So each organ has a unique identity and function and works together with other organs to live and grow as a human being.

Paul wrote to the Corinthians about the body of Christ, the church, and how each part of the body works together for the sake of the whole body. Jesus came to earth to redeem and restore people to their identity and function as children of God. Peter's identity was clarified by Jesus when Jesus said you are the rock, and upon this rock I will build my church. When Peter got a revelation of who Jesus was, then Jesus gave Peter a revelation of his identity. Just as God creates life in the mother's womb and establishes the identity and function of individual organs as well as the person as a whole, we find our identity, not by searching inwardly, but by a revelation of who Jesus is. The Holy Spirit then confirms our calling and election. Each part of the body of Christ has identity and function that, when operating properly, makes a healthy body of Christ.

A cancer can occur when just one cell loses its identity. It becomes less differentiated, that is to say, a cancerous liver cell does not look and behave so much like a liver cell any longer. This can occur from an injury of some sort to the DNA. It could be a mutation or an error in cell division. We know of some carcinogens that can increase the risk for cancer, such as cigarette smoking. There could be errors in the genetic code that are passed down from generation to generation. Many cancers have an increased occurrence in the family tree.

So cancer cells have a different appearance, when viewed under a microscope, compared to healthy, normal cells of the same organ. They do not look and function like normal healthy cells any longer. They have lost their identity to some degree.

Apoptosis

The 2nd characteristic of all cancer cells is that they do not die at their life expectancy. Apoptosis is a term used to describe programmed cell death. For example, red blood cells live about 120 days on average. The cells of the inner lining of the intestines last about five days. Built into the genetic code of each person's DNA is apoptosis, that is, an appointed lifespan for each of the various types of cells in the organs of the human being. Part of the loss of identity of a cancer cell is its programmed lifespan. So cancer cells may live shorter or longer than prescribed in the DNA code. Often there is an increased demand for these abnormal cells to grow and divide. This is termed a 'tumor burden' which may cause people to lose weight, become short of breath, and get fatigued.

Romans 11:29 states, "It is appointed unto man to die once, and after this comes judgment." This appointment for death is a result of our fallen nature into sin. God's righteous requirement for payment for sin is death. God's intent was never to fix or repair our human nature. The only answer for our old, sinful nature is death. If you are getting therapy from a Christian counselor who skips over this very foundational truth and attempts to rebuild and repair broken areas rather than take them to the cross where they have been crucified with Christ, this counsel and therapy could be said to be opposing God's plan. The first move for the human condition is to the cross where we encounter a merciful God. Then counseling, when built upon this truth, can be helpful.

The apostle Paul said in Colossians 3.3: "For you have died, and your life is hid with Christ in God." Paul viewed himself as one who had died and was now alive in Christ. The same is true for all believers. Because of the price paid by Jesus Christ on the cross, believers have passed from death into life and the old sinful nature within is crucified with Him. This becomes true when we place our trust in Him for salvation. It is a foundational, central theme in baptism. Romans 6 records that we are baptized into His death, so that we may then participate in His life.[2]

Just as death is essential for receiving the life of Jesus Christ, so also the programmed cell death of various cells in the organs of our body is necessary for maintaining bodily health.

Metastasis

Thirdly, cancer cells have the capability to spread to other parts of the body and reside elsewhere. This can happen through the blood stream, lymphatic flow, or by spreading directly to neighboring tissues. So a cancerous lung cell could spread to the liver and reside and grow there. This characterizes a more advanced staging of cancer. A metastatic cancer cell has spread to invade other organs and interrupt their function.

Cancer can begin with just one cell losing its identity, multiplying and growing, refusing to die, and spreading to other areas of the body.

As for the body of Christ, the church, it best functions when each part understands their calling and election. When each person in the body of Christ submits to Jesus, the head, and fulfills their role, cooperating with the others members of the body, then the body is healthy and productive. Conversely, when members of the body of Christ do not submit to the Head, attempt to reside and function outside of their calling and election, are at odds with other members, or simply not functioning or performing, this is an unhealthy and unproductive body.

> "Let no one disqualify you, insisting on self-abasement and worship of angels, taking his stand on visions, puffed up without reason by his sensuous mind, and not holding fast to the Head, from whom the whole body, nourished and knit together through its joints and ligaments, grows with a growth that is from God" Colossians 2:18-19.

How to Minister

How then can we speak to "this mountain" called cancer? We know that the name Jesus is greater than any other name. His name is above all other names including all the names of different kinds of cancer. So we can speak to the cancer, call it by name, and command it to leave in the name of Jesus. We are invoking the Name of Jesus over the name of the particular cancer. The greater Name of Jesus is authoritative. We can be more specific by speaking directly to the cancer cells, commanding them to stop growing and spreading, and commanding those abnormal cells to die in the name of Jesus.

Each type of cancer can have certain specific symptoms and complications. Address those particular "mountains" also. Bless the normal functioning cells. Speak to the person's immune system telling it to recognize and remove cancerous cells.

Chapter 22

Infectious Diseases

———————————————⋆———————————————

There are several types of infectious pathogens that can cause suffering: bacteria, viruses, fungi, yeast, protozoa, and helminths (worms).[1] Some of these organisms coexist with us in a symbiotic relationship.

Bacteria

Bacteria are single celled organisms with a cell membrane but without a nucleus or other organelles. Most antiseptics kill bacteria by destroying the membrane. When we learned more about the benefits of soap, alcohol based antiseptics, and antibiotics, for some time there was a belief that we could conquer bacteria once and for all time. We know now this is not possible. Moreover, it is really not desirable as bacteria play important roles in our lives.

Bacteria are almost everywhere on earth. They reside in the normal flora of our skin and gut. Bacteria on and in our bodies outnumber the number of cells in our body by a factor of ten. Some bacteria are beneficial; others can become pathologic causing infection. The vast majority of bacteria are rendered harmless by our immune system.

Bacteria cause disease by either adhering to or entering the cell or by delivering bacterial toxins. These induce responses directed against the bacteria. There may be purulence (pus), scarring, and hypersensitivity reactions. These responses themselves may cause additional tissue damage.

Common infections caused by bacteria include urinary tract infections, lower respiratory infections or pneumonia, skin infections such as cellulitis and cutaneous abscesses, and some upper respiratory infections. These can occur from exposure to someone else with infection or can arise from an overgrowth of bacterial flora.

Viruses

Most upper respiratory and gastrointestinal infections are caused from viruses. A virus is an obligate intracellular parasite; it can only function when it is inside a cell. A virus is made up of a segment of DNA or RNA inside a capsule. The DNA or RNA of the virus when inside of a cell takes command of some of the functions of the cell to replicate itself and spread out to infect other cells. A virus is really not alive so we cannot really kill a virus.

Each cell of our human body has a surface coating called the glycocalyx. Glycocalyx literally means "sugar coat". This sugar coat on the surface of the cells of our body recognizes certain minerals, vitamins, electrolytes, hormones, etc. and may allow these things to penetrate through the cell membrane. The glycocalyx may also reject certain items that are not needed or are harmful. The capsule of a virus has a similar appearance to some molecules that the cell would normally accept and thereby tricks the cell's glycocalyx to allow the virus inside the cell. Once inside the cell the virus uses the cell's resources to replicate itself. The only solution for a virus-infected cell is for that cell to die.

This battle against infection has insightful parallels with our battle against temptations and sin. A temptation has some kind of appeal and offers something of interest to us. Like a virus that deceives the cell membrane, a temptation can trick us into thinking that we can receive some kind of satisfaction by investing in its appeal. The longer we look at a tempting desire the more its appeal increases. If we invest ourselves in its appeal and act on that temptation, we have succumbed to it. Unless we repent and seek forgiveness, that sin and sinful nature will grow and ultimately produce death. "Each person is tempted when he is lured and enticed by his own desire. Then desire when it has conceived gives birth to sin; and sin when it is full-grown brings forth death" James 1:14-15.

To be tempted is not sin, but it becomes sin when we internalize and invest ourselves or take action on the temptation. Just as a virus infected cell must die, the only solution for sin is death. God never intended to fix or repair the sinful human being. His answer has always been death. God said to Adam and Eve that the day that they ate from the fruit of the tree of knowledge of good and evil, in that day they would surely die. The Hebrew text actually says, "Dying, you will die".[2] Sin has an immediate consequence and an ultimate result. The good news of the gospel is that God sent His own son Jesus Christ to die in place of our sins. He paid the price to set us free.

An infection from a virus, bacteria, or fungus can cause a fever. The fever is actually beneficial, though uncomfortable. A fever is good in that it revs up our metabolism and speeds up our immune response to battle the infection. The increased temperature also makes an unfavorable environment for many of these pathogens.

How to Minister

Jesus said, "You will say to this mountain, move from here to there, and it will move" Matthew 17:20. So with regard to infectious diseases, what is "this mountain"? How should you speak a word of command to minister healing to someone stricken with an infection? You can speak to the pathogen to die and to leave the person's body. You can rebuke the fever, as Jesus did, and drive out the infectious agent in the Name of Jesus.

"Mountain" in the Scripture has a demonstrative pronoun modifying it, namely the word "this". Jesus instructs us to be specific. You will say to THIS mountain. So if you happen to know the type of infection and where it is causing symptoms, you can be very specific in how you direct the word of command. For example, a person with strep throat has an infection caused by bacteria called Streptococcus. So you can command the Streptococcus bacteria to die and leave the sick person's body. You can also speak blessing to the immune system and loose or release it to attack the infection.

Chapter 23

Infirmities & Injuries

The term 'infirmity' is a biblical term. ἀσθένεια (*asthéneia*), in Greek, literally means weakness and loss of strength. It is a broad term that can describe loss of function due to a variety of causes. An infirmity can be the result of an injury, joint wear and tear from degenerative disease or overuse, or one of many diseases that can cause pain and weakness. In this section we will look at how to speak to this mountain, when it pertains to various injuries, weaknesses and pains.

These are very frequent complaints that involve joint aches and pains, muscle weakness and disability, and degenerative diseases. Neck and back pains are very common symptoms. Almost everybody will have at least one episode of significant back or neck pain at some time in life. Very often we become vulnerable to these symptoms because we expect much from our neck and back without conditioning and strengthening these muscles.

Regular exercise has many benefits including preventing neck and back injuries. Additionally, proper stretching and strengthening can bring relief to musculoskeletal injuries, including back and neck pain. These kinds of pains do serve a purpose. Pain is a language that various parts of our body use to communicate information to us about lifestyle, balance in life, and guarding an injured area.

Pain

Almost everybody has pain. Pain serves a purpose; it is usually not appropriate to completely get rid of pain. A significant problem has evolved in the effort to treat pain using medications. There are upwards of 15,000 deaths per year now in United States of America from combinations of medications, often including narcotics, used to treat chronic pain. You have heard of celebrities whose lives have tragically ended because of overdoses and mixtures of these kinds of medicines. There are countless others you do not hear about. It has become a big problem and is forcing doctors and the drug enforcement agency to change policies and standards of care for treating chronic pain. These medications can be beneficial initially in treating pain, but prolonged use can actually increase pain and create addiction and dependency on them.

I was recently on a medical mission to Columbia. Many people think of Columbia as one of the big sources of illegal drugs. We worked with people on an island near Cartagena. They worked hard and often complained of headaches, neck and back pain. They were very happy to have acetaminophen or ibuprofen to treat these pains. Contrast that clinics and emergency departments across our country where every day people check in expecting to receive strong narcotics for chronic pain. The longer these medicines are used, the more tolerant we become to them, and pain rebounds even more intensely, bringing a person to request more and more pain medicine.

In the emergency department where I work, we have now established a policy that we do not treat any chronic pain, headaches, or dental pain with narcotics. We will treat only with nonnarcotic options. If there is a new identifiable injury, such as a broken bone, we will use narcotic medicines as may be necessary. I recently spoke with one of the nurses who stated that, before this policy, she felt that her primary function was to give out pain medicine. At that time she was very seriously considering quitting her nursing work.

Pain also serves a purpose to point us to our Creator, to seek Him for healing. It can also serve as a marker to determine if a healing touch of God has occurred. Very often I ask people what symptoms they are currently experiencing. Then after ministering healing by

173

laying on of hands and word of command, I ask if any of these symptoms have resolved or improved. It is important to ask this before and after ministry because many times God's healing touch is so gentle that people may not realize their pain is improving or gone. Sometimes there is no change in pain, but a distinct awareness of God's healing touch such as warmth, a feeling of something like electrical energy, or a sensation of movement in certain parts of the body. The pain then resolves later as the cause of the pain is healed.

I experienced this myself many years ago. I had been spending lots of time reading, writing, and studying while in my seminary training. So I had acquired terrible neck pain. After learning about how to minister healing for this (explained later in this chapter), I felt movement in my neck and shoulders, but there was no relief of the pain. I knew with certainty that God's healing hand had touched me, but there was no change in the pain I was experiencing. So I simply began thanking God for this healing touch. Over the next day the pains in my neck were completely gone, and gone to this day. God corrected the underlying problem causing the pain, then over time the muscles, nerves, etc. began to relax and stop hurting.

Many times people requesting healing can demonstrate some kind of weakness, pain, or disability. It is a great testimony to the grace and power of God when those symptoms change or resolve. When symptoms are clarified before healing ministry occurs, God's healing touch is more readily identified. So often healing comes so quietly and simply that people may not even realize that there was a change unless you determine clearly the symptoms before and after a ministry encounter.

There are too many causes of weakness and injury for us to unpack here. There are, however, a few important general strategies that we should use when ministering to these types of matters.

When a person presents with back or neck pain it may be from an injury event, inflammatory causes, nerve impingement, muscle spasms, or other less common causes. Sometimes it becomes clear, as you discuss the nature of the neck and back pain, what is the underlying mechanism of pain. If so, you can address these specific matters as you lay hands on the person's neck or back.

Neck Pain

If a person has neck pain, I will often have them stretch their arms forward, with palms facing each other, but not touching. Then ask them to bring their hands together and look for any difference in the length of the arms. This is not an exact measurement. Sometimes it may be convenient to have this person lean back against a wall to remove some of the variability in making this assessment. If there is a difference in the length of the arms, (the arms may not actually be different in length, but this can demonstrate some asymmetry related to all of the structures in the neck and upper back and arms), I then have them continue to hold their arms extended without palms touching each other. I will often speak to the structures of the back and neck and arms to receive healing in Jesus name. I command the ligaments bones, tendons, and muscles to be in proper position. Then I command the short arm to grow out and become the same length as the other. I also commend the pain to leave in Jesus name.

Do this with your eyes open and watch what happens. Wait for a few minutes, while you keep your hand placed on the person's neck or back, and allow time for God's healing power to work. After a few minutes if nothing occurs, consider if there may be another mountain that may need to be addressed. If the person's neck pain is a result of a traumatic injury, it may be appropriate to drive away any spiritual forces that may have attached themselves to that traumatic injury.

Sometimes a person feels structures moving in their body. Other times there is no sensation of any change, even though the short arm may grow or adjust to the same length as the other arm. Sometimes the pain persists despite an adjustment that occurs. Again, pain is a symptom possibly pointing to some underlying source. This strategy involves speaking to this mountain to minister healing to the underlying cause of pain. Additionally, speak to the pain itself, commanding it to leave.

Back Pain

The same strategy can be performed when ministering healing to lower back, hip, and leg pains. You can check the length of a person's legs by sitting them up straight in a chair with the lower back and hips slid all the way back into the chair. As stated before, this is not a precise assessment. Changing position by rotating the hips or even turning the ankles may skew this measurement. Use a firm chair if available, one that does not have much of a cushion behind the person's lower back, in order to acquire a more accurate assessment of leg length.

Then you can reach down and take the ankles or heels in your hands and straighten the legs, looking at the heels of the shoes to assess symmetric leg length. You can also put your thumbs over the medial malleolus (the inner bump) of each ankle. Then use your thumbs to demonstrate to you, the person you are ministering to, and others gathered around, any difference in leg length.

Raising the legs up like this when in a sitting position is similar to a medical assessment maneuver called the 'straight leg raise'. Some people may have significant pain in the lower back when raising up either or both legs. It may be too painful for some to hold the legs in this position. This can be a clue that there may be a nerve impingement in the low back. As part of your ministry strategy you can speak to the impingement of these nerves and release them from pressure from surrounding structures, in particular, a herniated disc.

Some people with back, hip, and leg symptoms will have symmetric or equal leg length. For these people I let them sit comfortably while I place my hand on their lower back to release God's healing power. I ask the Holy Spirit to come upon them and within them and touch them with a healing touch. I then speak to the structures of the back commanding the bones, ligaments, nerves, tendons, and muscles to be in proper position and function. I speak to the pain and command it to leave in Jesus name.

If there is a difference in leg length of a half inch or more, this could be a cause or a symptom related to a person's low back, hip or leg pain or weakness. While holding their ankles in my hands with my thumbs over the bump of the inner aspect of each ankle, I ask the Holy Spirit to come and touch with healing power. Then I speak to the structures of the back as I just described. I address the bones, tendons, ligaments, muscles, and nerves to be in proper position and function in Jesus' Name. Then I speak to the short leg and command it to grow out and become the same length as the other. Sometimes an immediate change with observable movement may occur. Sometimes I patiently wait for several minutes. While waiting I often talk casually with the person about anything such as the weather or sports. Often I will use this time to instruct and describe various ways God's healing occurs. Sometimes we miss God's healing touch because we do not wait expectantly even just for a few minutes. During this time I consider again if there may be some other mountain that needs to be spoken to in Jesus' Name.

Degenerative Disease

Joint aches and pains of various locations including back and neck may be a result of degenerative disease,[1] occurring commonly in the latter half of life as our joints suffer from regular activity. Degenerative disease also has a genetic component, tending to run in families. Early degenerative disease can be a result of a prior injury. There are autoimmune diseases discussed in another chapter that can cause degenerative disease. Studies have shown that exercise can serve to protect the health of our joints. Other studies of showing exercise, especially heavy exercise, can contribute to degenerative disease.

All of us will have changes that occur as the years and decades pass. We cannot stop this process. Paul said, "Though our outer nature is wasting away, our inner nature is growing stronger every day" 2 Corinthians 4:16. We can make lifestyle choices to promote health. Nevertheless, the aches and pains of joints that have degraded can cause significant suffering and impaired mobility and function.

In general, degenerative diseases occur when the cushion of the joint wears down. When this cartilage degenerates, the space in the joint becomes more narrow and the ligaments stabilizing the joint can loosen. There are changes that occur in the synovial fluid that lubricates the joint. The bones at the joint can react by growing osteophytes–bony prominences at the edge of the joint. Consequently, there is often pain, decreased mobility, and increased instability. Knees and hips are common joints that degenerate. The back and neck can also degenerate, losing the protective cushion between the bones of the vertebrae.

So when ministering healing to those with degenerative joint pains and disability, I will often speak to the cushion of the joint to regenerate, speak to the synovial fluid to properly lubricate the joint, and command the pain to leave in Jesus' name.

Shoulder Pain

Most common causes of shoulder pain are a result of trauma or overuse injuries. Traumatic injuries include dislocation, separation, tendon injuries, and fractures. Overuse injuries include bursitis and rotator cuff tendinitis.

When ministering to someone with shoulder complaints, assess the range of motion and location of pain before ministering healing. Place a hand on the affected shoulder and ask the Holy Spirit to come and touch the person with His healing touch. Then speak to the shoulder to be healed in the Name of Jesus. Command the pain to leave. Speak to the shoulder for its range of motion to be restored to normal. If the underlying mechanism of pain and weakness is known, address that specifically. Then speak to the person and tell them to raise their arm up in the name of Jesus. Ask them to test it out to see if there is any change in pain and range of motion. You may keep a hand on the shoulder and talk about how God's healing touch can work instantly or over some time. You may have some casual conversation, all the while giving time for God's healing power to bring restoration.

A great visual testimony occurs when a person is able to raise up an arm that previously had restricted motion and was painful. It is very easy to observe a change in range of motion when ministering to a person's shoulder. Notice the extent of movement before speaking a word of command, then check it again after ministry. Such healings are an awesome demonstration of God's love, grace, and healing power. A shoulder healed by Jesus can provide visual evidence of the presence of God. Healings are a sign of the nearness of the kingdom of heaven. Such signs and wonders accompany and amplify the words of the gospel and bring people to reckon with their own lives before a loving and gracious God.

Trauma and Injuries

Accidents and injuries happen to everyone. A scar is a reminder of an injury and is a wonderful indicator of our bodies' God-given ability to repair itself. Jesus, the Son of God, was injured, beaten, and put to death on a cross. He was raised from the dead with scars on His hands, feet, and side as a result of human activities. When those who believe are taken up to heaven they are given a new body. Perhaps the only remnant of the old human nature yet in heaven is Jesus' scars on His hands, feet, and side.

God has created our bodies with an ability to repair themselves to a certain degree. An injury event causes the release of chemical messengers called cytokines. These cytokines signal the recruitment of increased blood flow to the area bringing macrophages to clean up debris, the immune system to fight off invasive pathogens, and nutrients for rebuilding damaged tissue, among many other amazing mechanisms of repair. This often causes swelling of the injured tissues. This inflammation is not all bad. It may restrict some range of motion, but it is necessary for cleaning and rebuilding an injured area.

A normal process of healing takes time. A healing touch of God may accelerate this process. Sometimes our bodies' natural healing occurs to a certain degree but not completely, with persistent symptoms months or years later. God's gift of healing brings restoration, reestablishment, and strengthening beyond the normal healing mechanisms He already created in each living thing.

I am grateful for the normal healing process that God has given to our bodies. And as you might surmise, as a medical doctor I do appreciate the various natural and medical remedies and treatments for all types of diseases and injuries. The Scripture says, "Seek first the kingdom of God, and His righteousness, and all these things will be added to you (Matthew 6.33). For me, if I have some pain or illness I do seek God first in prayer, but I do not wait too long to consider some acetaminophen or ibuprofen for relief if not improving. I do not have a conflict in my understanding of the Scriptures and God's healing power with my understanding of most of the natural, medical, and surgical options.

All things are possible with God. Let's not limit what He is able and willing to do. Once a woman came to me with a simple request.

She wanted her fingers back. She explained that she had crushed the ends of her fingers in a heavy 20,000 lb. press. She showed me her hand with her index, middle, and ring fingers all the same length as her little finger. To be honest with you, I did not have much expectation or faith for results. Nevertheless, I took her hand between my two hands and began to pray. She interrupted my prayer saying she could feel something was happening. So I held her hand with my index finger marking the ends of her fingers. There were about a dozen people watching as we saw her fingers grow back over the next couple minutes.

With God all things are possible. We, as members of His body the church, are the ones God chooses to bring blessings to others. If we had received comfort from God, then we are able to bring comfort to anyone in any affliction.[2] This holds true for any type of trauma and injury.

When ministering to ones who suffer under the effects of a traumatic injury, carefully listen to the guidance of the Holy Spirit as you hear from the person the basics of what happened and what symptoms yet remain. Remember that it may be helpful to bind and drive away any power assignment from the enemy that may have caused the injury event or holds a person in a diseased or injured condition. Then lay hands on the person and ask for the Holy Spirit to come and touch them with healing power. Then speak specifically to "this mountain", the pain and disability related to their injury.

Chapter 24

Endocrine Diseases

———————❖———————

I magine sitting at an intersection watching cars drive down the road. You are looking for a Maserati because you know that the driver of a Maserati has a message for you. You might see a million or more cars before you see a Maserati. When you recognize the car you are looking for, it triggers an emotional response inside you. You are happy to see what you were searching for and signal to the driver to stop to deliver his message. This scenario gives some insight into the incredible function of hormones serving as chemical messengers. A hormone circulating in the blood stream may occur as a one-in-a-million molecule.

Now imagine sitting at the same intersection again looking for a Maserati but this time with blinds over your eyes and plugs in your ears. Furthermore the driver of the Maserati will not be able to see you or hear you. So it is with hormones and their corollary receptors. Hormones and their receptors have an affinity toward one another, but neither have eyes or ears to find the other. Together with the nervous system, hormones serve to regulate the function of many organs and systems. These chemical messengers either stimulate or suppress activities in cells and organs by triggering action to maintain normalcy or homeostasis. This is another amazing detail of how fearfully and wonderfully we are made.

Hormones

The hormones elaborated by the endocrine glands interact with their target organs via cell receptors. The word 'hormone' is derived from Greek meaning 'to excite' or 'to stir up'. The endocrine system forms an important communication system that serves to regulate, integrate, and coordinate a variety of different physiologic processes falling into four areas: the digestion, utilization, and storage of nutrients; growth and development; ion and water metabolism; and reproductive function.[1]

A hormone molecule secreted into the blood is free to circulate and contact almost any cell in the body. However, only target cells, those cells that possess specific receptors for the hormone, will respond to that hormone. When a hormone binds to its receptor, biologic effects characteristic of that hormone are initiated.

Feedback regulation is an important part of endocrine function. The endocrine cell has the ability to sense the consequences of secretion of its hormone. This enables the endocrine cell to adjust its rate of hormone secretion to regulate the desired effect to maintain homeostasis. For example, insulin and glucagon are constantly regulating levels of glucose in the blood. Insulin functions to bring glucose out of the blood and into muscle or fat cells; glucagon does the opposite by raising levels of glucose in the blood.

There are many hormones circulating in our bodies. Some of them are better understood than others. There are likely other hormones yet to be discovered. More commonly known hormones include: thyroxin, thyroid stimulating hormone (TSH), insulin, glucagon, growth hormone, testosterone, estrogen, progesterone, prolactin, oxytocin, parathyroid hormone, serotonin, melatonin, epinephrine, dopamine, and erythropoietin. There are many others not listed here. These hormones originate in various endocrine glands and other non-endocrine organs such as the: hypothalamus, pituitary, thyroid gland, parathyroid glands, adrenal glands, pancreas, testes, ovaries, kidney, heart, stomach, and skin.

Some disorders related to the endocrine glands are common such as type 2 diabetes mellitus, gestational diabetes, thyroid disorders, and osteoporosis. Other less common endocrine related disorders include hyperparathyroidism, diabetes insipidus, hypopituitarism, Cushing's disease, polycystic ovary syndrome, growth disorders.

This is a very superficial description of very complicated disease states. Again, it's not necessary to know anything about these endocrine related disorders in order to minister God's healing power. This information is provided to give a strategy for ministry that is more specific. Despite their complexity it is rather simple to speak to 'this mountain' as it pertains to endocrine diseases. The underlying mechanism of pathology for all of these disorders is a disruption of the normal function of specific hormones and their receptors.

How to Minister

So how would one speak to 'this mountain' for someone with thyroid disease? There are different types of thyroid conditions, but in any of them one can speak to the thyroid to produce appropriate amounts of thyroxine. All of the many associated symptoms will resolve in time if thyroid hormone levels are proper. One can also speak to the various symptoms under which a person may be suffering.

Type 2 diabetes mellitus is a very common disease in our society. Being overweight with a sedentary lifestyle causes increased risk of this disease. Those who stay active and avoid becoming overweight will not likely contract this disease. It is a rather complicated condition involving many organs in the body. Simply stated, this disease is primarily caused by resistance to insulin. The receptors for the insulin hormone do not respond as they should to allow glucose to enter into the muscle or fat cells. This resistance to insulin causes the pancreas to produce higher levels of insulin to compensate for the receptor's resistance. As this disease progresses the pancreas becomes less able to produce these larger amounts of insulin and eventually will require exogenous injectable insulin medication. Type 2 diabetes mellitus is a condition that is related to the pancreas, liver, and kidneys. Prolonged high levels of blood glucose will cause neuropathy, retinopathy, vascular disease, and other consequences.

Type 1 and Type 2 diabetes mellitus are similar in that both have increased blood glucose levels that will eventually cause end organ damage (kidneys, nerves, vision, vasculature, etc). The difference between type 1 and 2 is the mechanism by which elevated blood glucose occurs. Type 1 is an autoimmune disease, discussed in the 'autoimmune disease' chapter, where high glucose levels occur because the immune system has destroyed the beta islet cells of the pancreas so that they do not produce insulin. Type 2, as discussed above, occurs when there is resistance to the effects of insulin. Type 1 has low levels of insulin and type 2 usually has high levels of insulin in the blood.

When ministering healing to someone with type 2 diabetes mellitus, it is appropriate to speak to the insulin resistance in the cell membranes to allow glucose to move from the blood stream into the cell. Speak to the liver commanding it to manage and metabolize glucose and lipids properly. Speak to the kidneys commanding them to regulate blood pressure and filter the blood properly. As for other endocrine diseases you can speak to the affected organs, glands, and hormones in similar fashion. Consulting a list of endocrine organs and associated hormones can assist you in crafting a way to speak to 'this mountain to move from here to there.'

Chapter 25

Behavioral Diseases

———————————————✦———————————————

'Behavioral health' is a term frequently used in health care systems. There are a very wide range of issues and diagnoses for which a person may engage in counseling and/or take certain medicines. These resources are used to treat disorders of mood, psychosis, addiction, phobias, among a large number of conditions related to mental and behavioral diseases.

Everyone knows someone who struggles with symptoms of depression and anxiety. Year after year, four or five of the top ten most prescribed medications are psychotropic medications, usually for depression and anxiety. Similarly everyone knows of someone who suffers with dementia or some other form of memory impairment. Additionally, everyone knows of people who struggle with cravings or addictions to tobacco products, alcohol, prescription or street drugs, and even food. Some of the more common diseases in this grouping include psychosis, depression, anxiety, panic disorder, bipolar disease, attention deficit hyperactivity disorder (ADHD), oppositional defiant disorder, eating disorders (anorexia nervosa, bulimia nervosa, binge eating), drug and alcohol abuse and addiction, psychosis, schizophrenia, paranoia, post-traumatic stress disorder (PTSD), obsessive compulsive disorder (OCD), dementia, developmental delay, autism, and tourette syndrome.

Behaviors and Disease

There are diseases that contribute to or cause certain behaviors, habits, or moods. Conversely, there are behaviors, habits, and moods that contribute to or cause certain diseases. These behavioral diseases have strong habitual and psychological components, but can also cause changes in physical health. These disorders are related to behaviors and choices, but there is also evidence of biochemical changes in the nervous system and neurotransmitters[1] that contribute to certain actions and behaviors. Every human resides in a body with a soul and spirit. A matter rooted in the soul can affect spirit and body. Bodily disease or harm affects one's soul and spirit. A wounded spirit causes symptoms to the body and soul.

We deserve the maladies that come as consequences of our own wrong behaviors or habits. We reap what we sow. Our wrong choices have consequences which can cause disease. If someone smokes long enough, we're not surprised when emphysema, lung cancer, stroke, heart disease, etc. occurs. Our choices sometimes cause irreversible consequences.

Certain bad habits such as smoking, gluttony, gambling, alcohol and other mood altering drugs bring consequences to people and others around them. There are a number of diseases that occur because of bad habits and choices. The fallen human nature can generate sickness and suffering that at times may be a reaping of the consequences of lifestyle choices.

Though we deserve these consequences as a result of our wrong choices and sins, Jesus took them upon Himself. Forgiveness and healing are gifts that we do not deserve, nor can we work for them. God's grace is sufficient for our salvation, but He does not remove all the consequences of sin and sickness. We may still have scars and memories reminding us. In the midst of this God promises to work all things together for good for those who love Him and are called according to His purpose.[2] In this life we do have hardships and suffering. These have a purpose to produce patience, character, perseverance, and hope.[3]

My grandfather smoked for 67 years of his life. He started smoking at age 14 and finally was able to quit at age 81. He suffered with emphysema because of his smoking. I repeatedly saw him turn blue, struggling for each breath when just trying to walk across the room. I had the privilege as a young man to lead him to the Lord. When he accepted Jesus into his heart, his spirit was made alive. At that time I also prayed for his breathing. He stated that he felt some improvement, but the damage had been done. He improved a little because he quit smoking. He also improved to a degree because of God's healing touch. He lived to be 91 years old. The last 10 years of his life were certainly better because he became a Christian and because he quit smoking. I do not remember seeing him turn blue anymore from lack of oxygen. Yet these years were not great as he continued to have limited mobility and lung function.

Our job as ones ministering healing is to freely give what we have freely received. It is not for us to act in judgment or withhold God's grace from anyone. God in His great wisdom, justice, and mercy will meet out those consequences.

This is the basic human problem, that we are slaves to sin and need a Savior. "For whatever overcomes a man, to that he is enslaved" 2 Peter 2:19. Each one of us has knowingly and unknowingly participated in harmful activities to ourselves and others.

"Do you not know that if you yield yourselves to any one as obedient slaves, you are slaves of the one whom you obey, either of sin, which leads to death, or of obedience, which leads to righteousness? But thanks be to God, that you were once slaves of sin have become obedient from the heart to the standard of teaching to which you were committed, and, having been set free from sin, have become slaves of righteousness" Romans 6:16-18.

"But then what return did you get from the things of which you are now ashamed? The end of those things is death. But now that you have been set free from sin and have become slaves of God, the return you get is sanctification and its end, eternal life. For the wages

of sin is death, but the free gift of God is eternal life
in Christ Jesus our Lord" Romans 6:21-23.

Though we all deserve the consequences of our wrong thoughts, actions, and words, the good news of the gospel is the freedom and imputed righteousness that comes through Jesus Christ for those who believe and receive Him.

Acquired Behavioral Diseases

Some behavioral diseases are acquired and others are innate or inborn. Acquired behavioral diseases may or may not be caused by wrong choices. These diseases are not present at birth or infancy, but occur later on. Some of these acquired diseases occur as a result of a person's choices. Alcohol dependence and addiction is viewed as a disease (there is evidence that a certain percentage of people have an innate predisposed to seek after and misuse alcohol and other drugs), but almost no one becomes addicted to alcohol without making a repeated choice to drink alcohol. An exception is fetal alcohol syndrome. A mother drinking enough alcohol while pregnant can cause physical and behavioral conditions in her child.

Other acquired behavioral diseases may not be caused by wrong choices. Alzheimer's dementia occurs in some elderly people. There is yet no statistically significant evidence of this condition occurring as a consequence of making wrong choices. Similarly, one who has paranoid schizophrenia will exhibit certain behaviors and beliefs. A downward social mobility occurs, that is, a decline in ability to function normally in society. However, there is no evidence of certain behaviors that cause this condition.

Innate Behavioral Diseases

There are also behavioral diseases that are inborn or innate. Though there may be related behaviors as a result of such disease conditions, there is no evidence of the disease state occurring as a result of wrong choices or behavior. Though disease entered into this world as a result of the fall of mankind into sin, we cannot assume that every behavioral disease is a consequence of behaviors. Childhood developmental delay, autism, and other congenital conditions can contribute to abnormal or wrong behaviors and may indicate therapy and medications, but there is no clear medical evidence of wrongdoing to bring on these inborn conditions.

Sins of the Parents

There are references in Scripture to a causal relationship between parent's choices and diseases of their offspring. God spoke to Moses about this in the giving of the Ten Commandments. "I the Lord your God am a jealous God, visiting the iniquity of the fathers upon the children to the third and fourth generation of those who hate me, but showing steadfast love to thousands of those who love me and keep my commandments" Exodus 20:5-6. The term 'ancestral bondage' refers to this visitation of the father's sins upon the children. There are ministry strategies to break these cords of iniquity involving confession, repentance, and forgiveness. The generational consequences of hateful sin are yet far less than the steadfast love shown to those who love God and keep His commandments. So mercy triumphs over judgment.

The prophets Jeremiah and Ezekiel spoke of the children tasting the bitter taste of their father's choices. "In those days they shall no longer say: 'The fathers have eaten sour grapes, and the children's teeth shall be set on edge.' But every one shall die for his own sin; each man who eats sour grapes, his teeth shall be set on edge" Jeremiah 31:29-30 (see also Ezekiel 18:2). Jeremiah foretold of the days when this causal relationship would no longer be stated. Ezekiel stated that that time had then come when this causal relationship would no longer be in force in Israel.

> "The soul that sins shall die. The son shall not suffer for the iniquity of the father, nor the father suffer for the iniquity of the son; the righteousness of the righteous shall be upon himself, and wickedness of the wicked shall be upon himself" Ezekiel 18:20.

Additionally, Jesus was asked about this matter by His disciples when they saw a man blind from birth. Jesus did not discount the possibility of the sins of the parents affecting children, but this particular man's blindness was not a result of his or his parent's sins.

> "As he passed by, he saw a man blind from his birth. And his disciples asked him, 'Rabbi, who sinned, this man or his parents, that he was born blind?' Jesus answered, 'It was not that this man sinned, or his parents, but that the works of God might be made manifest in him'" John 9:1-3.

As for sins of the parents visited upon and affecting their children, the blood of Christ has purchased freedom from ancestral bondage. This victory has been accomplished for us by Jesus' death on the cross and His work of redemption in those who receive Him and believe in Him. "You know that you were ransomed from the futile ways inherited from your fathers, not with perishable things such as silver or gold, but with the precious blood of Christ, like that of a lamb without blemish or spot" 1 Peter 1:18-19.

Repentance and Forgiveness

Will God give physical healing to one who is unrepentant? Does unrepentant, unforgiven sin always prevent or inhibit God's healing touch to the same physical body? There are stories of healing in Scripture where forgiveness happened first before physical healing. An example is the paralytic who was healed of his paralysis AFTER Jesus stated 'your sins are forgiven you' (see Luke 5:18-26). Instructions regarding healing ministry in the book of James teach us to confess sins to one another and pray for one another IN ORDER THAT you may be healed (James 5:14-16).

There are other instances recorded in Scripture where Jesus healed first and later addressed sin. When Jesus healed and fed the multitudes there was no mention of repentance and forgiveness as a necessity to receive these blessings. At times Jesus healed first then instructed the one healed to sin no more. Repentance and forgiveness, though connected to physical healing and always is a beneficial practice, is not a prerequisite for physical healing. Just as Christ died for us while we were yet sinners, He was whipped and those stripes brought healing to us also while we were yet sinners. Such undeserved grace and blessing brings about heartfelt contrition and a desire to serve and obey God. His kindness leads us to repentance.

Do you WANT to be healed?

> "Now there is in Jerusalem by the Sheep Gate a pool, in Hebrew called Bethzatha, which has five porticoes. In these lay a multitude of invalids, blind, lame, paralyzed. One man was there, who had been ill for thirty-eight years. When Jesus saw him and knew that he had been lying there a long time, he said to him, 'Do you want to be healed?' The sick man answered him, 'Sir, I have no man to put me into the pool when the water is troubled, and while I am going another steps down before me.' Jesus said to him, 'Rise, take up your pallet, and walk.' And at once the man was healed, and he took up his pallet and walked ... Afterward, Jesus found him in the temple, and said to him, 'See, you are well! Sin no more, that nothing worse befall you'" John 5:.2-9, 14.

Do you want to be healed? You would think the obvious answer was 'yes'. Jesus asked him this question about his physical condition, but the question was directed at his will, thoughts, and beliefs. Some people do not want to be healed perhaps because of some of the responsibilities then required of them. The paralyzed man did not give a direct answer, but inferred that he wanted to be healed. His only hope was to be taken into the waters of the pool when they were stirred up, indicating a belief that there was healing power when this occurred. This was enough of a 'yes' answer for Jesus who then healed him. Jesus told him LATER to sin no more, lest nothing worse should befall him. He healed him first, and then spoke to his choices in life.

Most of us would consider paralysis for 38 years to be a very unfortunate condition. This man was unable to move on his own. He always required someone else to help him. Day after day for decades his life was same. His physical body was paralyzed. His heritage, identity, and destiny were also paralyzed. However, Jesus stated there was something worse than this. Jesus states here that unrepentant sin has worse consequences. "Sin no more, that nothing worse befall you" John 5:14. Jesus indicates that the wages of sin are worse than a lifetime of paralysis.

How to Minister

When someone repeatedly chooses things that are harmful and contracts a disease, do we minister healing when the disease state is a consequence of their own behaviors? If someone calls upon the church for healing, we should minister such as instructed in the book of James. "If ANYONE is sick, let them call upon the elders of the church and let them pray over him" James 5:14. The instructions here to the elders of the church are to pray the prayer of faith. There were no qualifications or requirements for this prayer ministry except for the sick person simply to come and call upon the elders of the church. The next verses then exhort us to confess sins to one another in order to be healed. I always pray for any sick person who asks.

How do we minister healing to this great variety of behavioral diseases? These diseases cannot be described by a single mechanism of disease. Many of these types of conditions have no obvious cause. A human being is made up of a body, a mind, a will, emotions, and a spirit. These all interact with one another in very complex and individual functions and expressions. Each person has an inherited personality given by God and an acquired personality derived from perspectives, conclusions, and belief systems that interpret life experiences. So there is great variety in a person's thoughts, emotions, experiences, and beliefs.

In every healing ministry encounter, it is best to listen to the guidance of the Holy Spirit and the Word of God. The gift of discernment and words of knowledge and wisdom are especially helpful in ministering to behavioral diseases. Don't forget the great battle in our minds. Don't disregard the spiritual battle in which we are engaged. Speak authoritatively to unseen strongholds and power assignments that may be holding a person captive to the particular disease or condition.

Lead them to the Lord in repentance, being careful not to blame or accuse of wrong behaviors. Ask the person seeking healing if there is any sin that needs confessiion and repentance. They can be led in a prayer that gives opportunity for silent or verbal confession and repentance.

Ask for the power of the Holy Spirit to come upon them. Bind the powers of the enemy and the symptoms of the disease and drive these out in the name of Jesus. Break any possible ancestral roots that may be connected to the behavioral disease. Bind the power of any harmful habits that may be involved. Pray for a way of escape from temptation as promised in 1 Corinthians: "No temptation has overtaken you that is not common to man. God is faithful, and he will not let you be tempted beyond your strength, but with the temptation will also provide the way of escape, that you may be able to endure it" 1 Corinthians 10:13. Often there is need for inner healing of emotional wounds, wounds of the soul and spirit that are crying out causing internal pain. There are wounds of feeling rejected by others that may serve to perpetuate various symptoms, behaviors, and beliefs that are harmful.

After leading in the above, address the symptoms by word of command. Speak to the organs affected by the disease. Seek understanding from reputable medical sources what are the primary causes and effects of the specific behavioral disease, if known. Then consider how to speak to 'this mountain,' and how to tell it to move. Then do as the Scripture says. Say to this mountain, 'move from here to there.'

There was a young mother with three children who came repeatedly to the emergency department. She was addicted to methamphetamines. It happened, by divine appointment, that each of the five times she came for help, I was the physician that saw her and treated her. At her fifth visit, it seemed to me she was finally completely honest and seeking for help. (So often those with addictions have trouble telling the truth.) She stated she had been reading a Bible and went to church a few times. I took the opportunity to explain to her that my first priority there was to be her medical doctor and provide appropriate care. I also explained that I was a Pastor and with her permission I took time to explain the good news of the gospel. I asked her if she was assured of her salvation. She had never asked Jesus into her heart and life; she was unsure of her standing before God. I led her in a prayer to invite Jesus into her life, forgive her of her sins, and deliver her from her addiction. That was the last time I saw her. I do not know what happened with her. Though I cannot prove it, I believe she was set free from her addiction to methamphetamines, seeing that she sincerely, honestly, and humbly gave her life to Jesus Christ.

Chapter 26

Other Diseases

The diseases and conditions discussed in previous chapters are grouped in categories that have similar mechanisms of pathology. The descriptions of these diseases in this book are over-simplified and not complete. Each disease has its unique features and characteristics. Understanding the generalized mechanisms of these diseases in their groupings is by no means a sufficient understanding of any of the diseases discussed. The groupings of diseases according to their primary mechanism of pathology are discussed solely for the purposes of understanding how one might speak to 'this mountain, telling it to move from here to there.' It is faith in Jesus and His word that ministers healing to every disease and every infirmity. It is not mandatory to understand these mechanisms of disease, but such understanding aids in an effort to speak specifically to 'this mountain' as Jesus instructs in the Word of God.

There are many diseases that have not been mentioned or discussed in the previous chapters. There are far too many diseases to address specifically in this book. Most of the ones not mentioned are not very common. The mechanisms of these diseases, if known, can be understood by searching for appropriate scientific literature or discussing them with a medical doctor. This research can be simple and superficial with the primary purpose to find what is 'this mountain' and where the 'here and there' is with respect to speaking to the mountain of a specific disease.

There are some rather common diseases that not discussed in the previous chapters. These diseases have unique or poorly understood mechanisms of pathology. This chapter is devoted to a brief discussion of some of these diseases that do not readily fit into the categories of mechanism of disease previously discussed. These are presented below in alphabetical order.

Fibromyalgia

Fibromyalgia is a syndrome or a set of symptoms that commonly occur together. Fibromyalgia is a combination of anxiety or depression, decreased pain threshold or tender points, fatigue, and widespread pain. Women are much more likely to have fibromyalgia symptoms. They are ten times more likely than men to acquire this disease. There are no reliable tests to confirm this diagnosis. So it is a clinical diagnosis, that is, a diagnosis is made on the presence of typical symptoms.

Fibromyalgia (fibro – myo – algia) literally means 'muscle fiber pain.' However, there is no evidence of pathology in the muscle fibers of those with symptoms of fibromyalgia. So the disease name is a misnomer. It is commonly believed that fibromyalgia has to do with the central nervous system.

Studies have been performed on healthy people to examine symptoms that occur when sleep deprived. After three days of no sleep or very little sleep, these otherwise healthy individuals all developed symptoms of fibromyalgia syndrome. The conditioned athletes that were studied developed fibromyalgia symptoms after four days of no sleep. Often those with fibromyalgia have insomnia; every person I know who has this syndrome reports trouble sleeping. Symptoms improve with better sleep and intense aerobic exercise at least two or three times a week. It's best to avoid pain medications, especially narcotics, as tolerance and dependency are likely.

When ministering to those with fibromyalgia, it is appropriate to address sleep. You can speak to the reticular activating system in the brain which controls wakefulness and sleep-wake transitions. You can also speak to the pain directly, commanding it to leave. It is reasonable to consider that this pain points to some cause. It may be insightful to ask those with fibromyalgia when the symptoms started and if there were circumstances that were traumatic around that time. It can be that a person's soul or spirit is troubled and the body manifests symptoms of this. Often it is like peeling layers of an onion to get to the core issues.

Gout[1]

Gout is a type of arthritis that causes sudden burning pain, stiffness, and swelling in a joint. This is usually in a big toe, but it can be any joint. Gout occurs more often in men. It is caused by too much uric acid in the blood. This occurs because of a deficiency of an enzyme called hypozanthine which breaks down purines to be excreted in the urine. High levels of uric acid in the blood can cause crystals to form in a joint. Chances of gout are higher in ones who are overweight, drink too much alcohol, or eat too much meat and fish which have high levels of purines. Some medications can trigger gout symptoms.

Prevention of a gout attack involves limiting offensive foods. A list of these foods and drinks can easily be acquired at a reputable medical website. Medical treatment of a gout attack often includes corticosteroids or non-steroidal anti-inflammatory drugs.

When ministering to an acute gout attack, it is appropriate to speak to the hypozanthine enzyme levels to increase and the uric acid levels in the blood to decrease. You can speak to the crystals that have formed in the joint to leave or dissolve. You can also command the pain to leave.

Headaches

There are several types of headaches that are common. A migraine headache often includes nausea, vomiting, and sensitivity to light and sound. Migraine headaches are not well understood. They may be caused by imbalances in brain chemicals called neurotransmitters. There seems to be a vascular component to this type of headache where blood vessels in the brain spasm and dilate. A tension headache is usually in the posterior occipital region of the head and often includes some neck pain. Sinus headaches occur because of fluid or pressure in the various sinuses in the head and face. This may occur as a result of sinus infection or allergy symptoms.

When ministering healing to someone with a headache, it may be helpful if it is possible to distinguish the type of headache as listed in the above paragraph. As you speak to headaches, you should command the pain to leave in the name of Jesus. You may acquire some insight where it can be appropriate to speak to the sinuses (sinus headache), blood vessels and neurotransmitters in the brain (migraine), or neck stiffness (tension headache). A tension headache may arise out of problems with the neck or back which can be addressed as discussed in the chapter entitled 'Infirmities and Injuries.'

Heart Diseases[2]
Dysrhythmias

Each cardiac muscle cell or myocyte has a characteristic called automaticity. This means that a cardiac cell has an innate ability to contract without external stimuli. There are various rhythm conditions of the heart that involve an alteration or disruption of the normal electrical flow[3] that causes the heart to squeeze out blood efficiently. Together these are called dysrhythmias. A person with a dysrhythmia may feel palpitations, lightheadedness, and shortness of breath among other symptoms. Examples of dysrhythmias include Premature Ventricular Contractions (PVCs), Premature Atrial Contractions (PACs), Supraventricular Tachycardia (SVT), and Atrial Fibrillation.

Premature contractions (PVCs and PACs) and Supraventricular Tachycardias occur because the heart is excitable. Caffeine use can increase occurrence of these conditions. PVCs and PACs are rather common. They do not cause concern unless they happen frequently (every other beat) or if they occur with other more troubling cardiac conditions. SVT is a fast heart rate (140 beats per minute and faster) at rest. This can occur intermittently for seconds or persist for hours or days. SVT occurs when a different part of the atria of the heart sets a faster pace and overrules the normal pacing of the sinoatrial node.

Atrial fibrillation is common in senior citizens (10-30%) and can be managed with rate controlling and anticoagulant medications. Here the cells of the atria are contracting without any organization. They are quivering or fibrillating but not effectively pumping blood into the ventricles. This is an irregularly irregular rhythm as the ventricles set the pace and rhythm of the heart. There are some various causes of AF but most often the cause is unknown.

When ministering to someone with these dysrhythmias, speak to the rhythm function of the heart. Speak to the heart muscle cells telling them to function in an organized contraction and to follow the pacing set forth by the sinoatrial node.

Ischemic Heart Disease

Ischemia occurs when there is an imbalance between supply and demand of the heart for oxygenated blood. This most commonly occurs with narrowing of the coronary vessels which perfuse the heart. These vessels can become narrow and have decreased blood flow potential because of atherosclerosis and cholesterol plaques. When the demand for oxygen and nutrients exceed the vessel's ability to supply these resources, a person will have symptoms of angina.[4] If supply and demand are not reconciled, a myocardial infarction (heart attack) may occur causing death to part of the muscle wall of the heart.

When ministering to someone with ischemic heart disease, speak to the coronary vessels to open, command the cholesterol plaques and atherosclerotic changes of the vessels to diminish.

Congestive Heart Failure

Congestive heart failure (CHF) occurs when there is impaired function of the heart, rendering it unable to maintain sufficient output of blood for the metabolic requirements of the tissues. Heart failure does not mean that the heart has stopped working; it signifies a heart whose pump function is decreased. This can cause the heart to remodel by stretching to hold more blood or the heart may become more stiff and thickened. The kidneys may respond by causing the body to retain fluid which builds up in the feet and legs, arms, and lungs so that the body becomes congested. CHF can be caused by ischemic heart disease, a heart attack, cardiomyopathy[5], or conditions that overwork the heart.[6] Symptoms often include shortness of breath with exertion, lightheadedness and fatigue.

To minister to CHF, you can speak to the heart to pump normally and speak to the fluid retention to return to normal. If the particular cause of CHF is known, this can be addressed specifically.

Hypertension[7]

There are various causes of hypertension, commonly referred to as high blood pressure. Most common is essential hypertension which is a relatively slow increase of blood pressure over time. Hypertension can be a consequence of many factors, including an adjustment of the regulatory feedback mechanisms. The kidneys, vascular tone (increased stiffness of the blood vessels), the sympathetic nervous system[8], along with other factors, contribute to changes in blood pressure.

High blood pressure usually does not cause symptoms, but untreated hypertension over time poses significant risks for heart disease, stroke, heart failure, peripheral vascular disease, vision loss, and kidney disease. Everyone's blood pressure will fluctuate according to various internal and external factors. These fluctuations are not hypertension. Hypertension is diagnosed and treated when at least three readings, measured when feeling normal, are elevated over at least two weeks.

For essential hypertension, it is more difficult to identify a single or primary cause and therefore it is more challenging to identify the 'mountain' that needs to 'move from here to there.' By definition, those with hypertension have increased blood pressure. So a believer can speak to the blood pressure itself, telling it to reduce to normal levels. You can say, "In the name of Jesus, I command the various components involved in regulating blood pressure to function properly and restore normal, healthy blood pressure levels.

Irritable Bowel Syndrome

Irritable Bowel Syndrome (IBS) is a group of symptoms involving abdominal pain and changes in patterns of bowel movements which may include diarrhea or constipation. There is no known underlying cause. Often IBS is associated with anxiety, depression, and chronic fatigue syndrome. Diagnosis of IBS is clinical, based on signs and symptoms in the absence of worrisome features. There are no labs or imaging studies that are conclusive for diagnosing IBS. Causes of IBS are not clear so there are many theories of the mechanisms of this condition, including gut-brain axis problems, bacteria overgrowth in the small intestine, food sensitivities, and gut motility problems.

When ministering to someone with IBS, it is tempting to suggest diet or lifestyle changes. Though these can be helpful, it is best to avoid this discussion (leaving it to the nutritionists and other experts) and bring the focus to Jesus and His word. Speak to the bowels commanding them to function properly. Command the spasms to relax. Speak to the muscles of the bowel to function in normal peristaltic manners.

Seizures

There are different types of seizures, but all types involve a disruption in the brain's natural circuitry. There are two broad categories of seizure types: generalized and partial. Generalized seizures are caused by electrical impulses throughout the entire brain. Partial seizures occur from electrical impulses in a relatively small part of the brain.

Seizures can occur because of several possible causes: genetics, a change in the structure of the brain, severe head injury, brain infection or disease, stroke, drug use, or lack of oxygen. Some seizures are provoked, that is, they occur as a result of a fever, drugs, or head trauma. This is not epilepsy which is a condition for which no cause is typically found.

When ministering to someone with seizures, speak to the brain telling it to stop producing excessive electrical impulses. If the type of seizure is known, especially if it is a provoked seizure, you may also speak to what caused the seizure, binding its power and consequences in the name of Jesus.

Stones

Stones can form in various parts of the body. There are kidney stones in the urinary tract, gall stones in the gall bladder, and canaliths in the vestibular system of the inner ear. The presence of these stones in their various places may not cause any problems or symptoms. Symptoms arise when these various stones move into nearby structures. Kidney stones can cause severe pain when moving down along the urinary tract. Gallstones can cause pain when blocking the flow of bile from the gall bladder into the common bile duct. Canaliths cause vertigo symptoms when they move into the semi-circular canals of the vestibular system.

When ministering to someone with these types of stones, speak to the stones telling them to dissolve or move. Issue a command to kidney stones to pass through the ureter to the bladder. Command gall stones to move back into the gall bladder or pass through the common bile duct to the duodenum. For both of these conditions, command the pain to be gone in the name of Jesus. Command canaliths to move out of the semi-circular canals back into the utricle (the sac of fluid that conjoins the canals). When addressing these stones, you could be truly speaking to this (very small) mountain, just one or a few stones, to move from here to there.

Vascular Diseases

There are diseases of the blood vessels including arteriosclerosis, peripheral vascular disease, and thrombotic events, coronary artery disease, and cerebral vascular disease. These diseases occur when inflammatory responses cause a thickening of the vessel wall and the formation of plaques. This can restrict blood flow causing a decrease of oxygen and nutrient supply to various tissues. A plaque can rupture causing the formation of a clot which can completely occlude the vessel. These conditions can arise because of genetic factors along with persistent elevations of blood pressure, cholesterol, and blood glucose. Smoking and lack of exercise also contribute to vascular disease. Vascular disease develops slowly under the influence of the above listed factors.

As with most of the diseases discussed in this chapter, there are many factors and conditions that cause vascular diseases. When the mechanisms of disease are unclear or multifactorial, a word of command can be directed to the symptoms themselves. So for vascular diseases you can speak to the thickened vessels to return to proper size and function. Speak to the vessels to allow normal flow of blood to the tissues.

Other Diseases and Conditions

For each disease state, what is the specific mountain that can be spoken to? What it is that needs to move from here to there? Where is 'here' and where is 'there' when speaking authoritatively to diseases and infirmities? The mechanisms of diseases vary with each disease. We can sometimes identify these 'mountains' when in a ministry encounter. If the underlying mechanism is not identifiable, we can always address the symptoms themselves.

For example, a man who complains of pain throughout his whole body may be suffering from one of many different causes of his pain. It is not clear what is causing his pain, so speak to the pain itself. His pain is the 'mountain' that can be addressed. The Holy Spirit may give a specific word of wisdom regarding the underlying cause of his pain. You should pursue these promptings, but avoid throwing commands at random 'mountains' hoping that something will respond.

A person seeking healing may come to you stating he has some disease or condition for which you do not know the underlying cause. For example, if a man comes requesting healing for Hirschsprung's disease or Castleman's disease, you will probably not know what symptoms are involved or what causes them. Many times the person seeking healing will be able to give some insight as to what causes his symptoms. Certainly he will be able to state what symptoms he experiences. This can guide you in speaking to 'this mountain' and what needs to move from here to there.

Section 4

USE YOUR AUTHORITY

F ew believers understand their authority in Christ. Of the ones who understand this measure of faith given to them by God, few are using it. Some of those who know their authority as believers are misusing it at times. To have mustard seed faith, the faith of the Centurion, is to know and use wisely the authority given by God.

This last section attends to strategies for a believer to use the authority given by God for the purposes of advancing God's kingdom. Consideration is given to proper attitudes and usage of this authority.

Chapter 27

Use Your Authority

One who studies the strategies and plans of woodworking is in a much better position to build items from wood successfully and to avoid injury with using power tools, but this person is not a woodworker until actually using the tools and building items with wood. One can study the art of cooking and watch TV shows and videos which teach how to cook all sorts of foods, but this person is not a cook or chef unless he actually prepares food himself. One who learns the language of music notation and studies the physics involved in what makes a trumpeter able to play each note is not a himself trumpeter until actually playing the trumpet skillfully. There are abundant similar illustrations that indicate the importance of knowing something. Yet this knowledge is incomplete without doing and practicing to acquire a certain related skill.

In the sport of baseball, those who lead in hitting home runs acquire this position by countless hours of practice and many failures at the plate. Home run leaders are often also strike out leaders. Even at the prime of performance, most of the time at the plate they do not hit a home run. What occurs most often is a failure to arrive on base. A very good batting average of 0.350 indicates two out of three of the 'at bats' are without a hit. Still these athletes face the pitcher each time with knowledge, experience, and faith that they can hit a home run or get on base one somehow.

The first time a believer uses his authority in Christ to speak a word of command for healing may not bring about a spectacular "home run" miracle. God looks for those who are faithful in little. It is best to start with little and save raising the dead for a little later. Over time and practice God will then set over much. Yet I have seen instant healings happen repeatedly when young believers are discipled and encouraged in a context of faith.

For many years I had the duty and pleasure to teach 8th grade students on Wednesday evenings. Each year I devoted at least one session to disciple them about God's will to heal and how to minister healing. I taught briefly just a few of the concepts about speaking a word of command to 'this mountain.' After asking who simply believed these words from Scripture, I selected a couple of them to minister healing in front of the others. Then I sought out anyone who had a headache or some other source of pain. Every year without exception someone received healing as these 8th grade students ministered to each other.

It was very mechanical, that is, they were not experienced. I gave step by step instructions: place your hand on the person's head; now say, 'In the name of Jesus, I command this headache (or other source of pain) to leave now.' I often had to repeat these simple instructions because they had never done this or spoken like this. It seems God is eager to demonstrate Himself to us and through us when we know and use our authority in Christ. We do not need to be eloquent or deliver a long prayer. It also seems God is pleased to demonstrate His kingdom in a public setting. He loves to show Himself in such signs and wonders as others are watching.

We gain confidence with instruction and teaching about certain tools and skills. Using those tools repeatedly brings us to become skilled and gain more confidence. Those who excel in knowledge, experience, and skill and are able to instruct others are said to be an authority in that realm. These people become an authority by virtue of knowledge, experience, and skill that comes by practice and over time. This parallels the New Testament concept and process of discipleship. To make disciples of all nations involves teaching each one to observe and obey what Jesus taught His disciples.

Do The Word

Faith comes by hearing and hearing by the Word of God. Those who hear the Word of God are able to have increased faith as a result of such hearing. Those who hear the Word of God and do what it says will be blessed. The epistle of James reports that faith apart from works is nothing; we show our faith by our works. When someone hears but does not do the Word, the Scriptures state this causes self-deception. Those who only hear and do not put the Word of God into practice will sooner or later be self-deceived.

> "But be doers of the word, not hearers only, deceiving yourselves. For if any one is a hearer of the word and not a doer, he is like a man who observes his natural face in a mirror; for he observes himself and goes away and at once forgets what he was like. But he who looks into the perfect law, the law of liberty, and perseveres, being no hearer that forgets but a doer that acts, he shall be blessed in his doing" James 1:22-25.

I envision a church as a place where the knowledge and the use of a believer's authority is taught, demonstrated, and practiced in a comfortable, non-threatening environment, a place where the great commission is carried out, to make disciples, teaching them to observe what Jesus taught His disciples, a place where the opportunity exists to try out the Word of God by doing what it says.

Most Christians do not really know and use their authority in Christ, resulting in a decrease in faith. Over time, one begins to question whether God does these works any longer, a type of self-deception. Faith grows when Jesus' authority is understood; faith grows further when believers understand and properly employ their authority.

Measure of Faith

Do your ministry according to the measure of faith given to you, according to the measure of authority given to you. The Centurion did not think of himself more highly (or lowly) than he ought. He showed sober judgment regarding himself and his position in the army. He understood the measure of faith and authority given to him and he functioned within that measure.

> "For by the grace given to me I bid every one among you not to think of himself more highly than he ought to think, but to think with sober judgment, each according to the measure of faith which God has assigned him. For as in one body we have many members, and all the members do not have the same function, so we, though many, are one body in Christ, and individually members one of another. Having gifts that differ according to the grace given to us, let us use them: if prophecy, in proportion to our faith; if service, in our serving; he who teaches, in his teaching; he who exhorts, in his exhortation; he who contributes, in liberality he who gives aid, with zeal; he who does acts of mercy, with cheerfulness" Romans 12:3-8.

So begin by using your gifts within the measure of faith and authority given to you. Don't start with raising the dead; rather start with using your authority over a headache or other aches and pains. When you are faithful in little, God will soon place you over much. Be persistent despite lack of results. Keep doing the Word of God. I have shared many stories of some of the more remarkable healings I have seen. I have seen the Lord Jesus do many other healings that are less spectacular. There are countless numbers of people that I laid hands on and spoke a word to this mountain that did not have any improvement and were not healed. Some of them died from their disease. Yet I keep doing the Word of God and I am still growing in faith. "Therefore having this ministry by the mercy of God, we do not lose heart" 2 Corinthians 4.1.

Let the Power Out

There are numerous ways that Jesus released power for healing and deliverance. Most commonly He spoke words and touched others. Word of command and laying on hands or touch were the most common ways Jesus and His disciples ministered to others. There were other means of grace, but these strategies are where we should begin to use our authority and release the power within us believers.

This is a great challenge for the church. The same power that raised Jesus from the dead dwells in believers who invite Jesus into their lives and are filled with the Holy Spirit. This power is present within believers but is hidden and not so apparent until we learn to let it out. We learn best how to let this power out by watching others who are functioning with understanding of their authority and appropriately use their authority in Christ. Look for opportunities to come alongside such people and join with them in ministering healing to others. Such mustard seed faith is more caught than taught.

Say to the Mountain

Just knowing your authority as a believer in Jesus, though it brings increased faith, does not bring results until one's authority is employed, used, or enacted according to God's will. Jesus said, "YOU will say to this mountain, 'move from here to there,' and it will obey YOU." Many people might ask God to move the mountain, but this is not what Jesus said we should do. He stated that WE should speak to the mountain. Some might argue with this and say, 'all things are possible with you, God, you move the mountain, we cannot.' Jesus is saying, 'I have given you authority, now you speak to the mountain.'

We might be reluctant to understand and function within our position before God. We may be thinking more lowly of ourselves than we ought, not understanding that believers are seated with Christ. The Centurion understood his position in the army and Jesus called that great faith. Nevertheless, understanding only is not enough. We must identify the mountain that we have authority over and simply speak to it. The Centurion spoke to those under his command, saying "come, go, and do this." It was not enough simply to have the authority. He used it appropriately to those under his command, and they obeyed. Jesus called this great faith.

God called Moses to lead the Hebrew people. God gave Moses a rod as a tool for God's power to be released. When Moses stretched the rod of God over the sea, the waters parted. When Moses struck the rock with the rod of God, water came forth from the rock. Moses had authority from God to lead the people and use the rod of God. God's power was released when Moses used the rod of God. We are given a 'rod of God'. When believers speak in the name of Jesus to this mountain, a 'rod of God' is wielded to advance His kingdom.

Jesus said that it is better that He goes back to His Father so that the Holy Spirit would come and perform greater works than Jesus did. The church, now the body of Christ, has this great power dwelling within each believer. Let's learn to let this power out according to the very clear instructions in the Scriptures how to release God's power for advancing His kingdom in accomplishing His will.

Touch and Lay Hands On

A touch can be a soothing gesture. When one rests a hand on another, there is a connection that occurs. It can be a caring, comforting maneuver. When a person reaches out to touch another person, the attention of that person is garnered. A touch penetrates a person's personal space.

God has ordained that a touch and laying on hands are also means by which His grace and power move from one person to another. When believers lay hands on another person in the name of Jesus, power goes forth to bless, comfort, and heal. Laying on of hands in prayer is a means by which gifts are imparted. The filling and empowering of the Holy Spirit often occurs in the context of laying on of hands. "Hence I remind you to rekindle the gift of God that is within you through the laying on of my hands" 2 Timothy 1:6.

Touch and laying on of hands is a mechanism Jesus used to minister to others. Sometimes Jesus simply touched people without saying any words and they were healed as power went forth through His touch.

> "And these signs will accompany those who believer: in my name they will cast out demons; they will speak in new tongues; they will pick up serpents, and if they drink any deadly thing, it will not hurt them; they will lay their hands on the sick, and they will recover" Mark 16:17-18.

> "And a leper came to him beseeching him, and kneeling said to him, 'If you will, you can make me clean.' Moved with pity, he stretched out his hand and touched him, and said to him, 'I will; be clean.' And immediately the leprosy left him, and he was made clean" Mark 1:40-42.

Faith in Action

Faith is not so much something you have as it is something you do. One can believe that a chair will hold a person up if it is sat upon. It takes faith to actually sit in the chair. This is what the book of James is talking about when he says, "Show me your faith by your works." Jesus said if you have faith as a grain of mustard seed, you will say... . Faith involves action. The Centurion also understood faith in this way.

There are times recorded in the Old and New Testaments when people were told to do something. When they obeyed, healing and miracles occurred. These occurred over some time and were dependent upon following the orders given. Faith means both 'obedience' and 'faith'. Healing happened because a person heard the word and did what was told.

Examples of faith in action:

- Go and show yourself to the priests.
  > "And as he entered a village, he was met by ten lepers, who stood at a distance and lifted up their

213

voices and said, 'Jesus, Master, have mercy on us.' When he saw them he said to them, 'Go and show yourselves to the priests.' And as they went they were cleansed" Luke 17:2-14.

- **Go wash in the Pool of Siloam.**

  "As he passed by, he saw a man blind from his birth. And his disciples asked him, 'Rabbi, who sinned, this man or his parents, that he was born blind?' Jesus answered, 'It was not that this man sinned, or his parents, but that the works of God might be made manifest in him. We must work the works of him who sent me, while it is day; night comes, when no one can work. As long as I am in the world, I am the light of the world.' As he said this, he spat on the ground and made clay of the spittle and anointed the man's eyes with the clay, saying to him, 'Go, wash in the pool of Siloam' (which means Sent). So he went and washed and came back seeing." John 9:1-7.

- Naaman, the Syrian commander, came to Elisha to be healed. Elisha did not even come out to see this great commander, but told him to wash in the muddy Jordan River waters. Naaman was expecting some great fanfare and turned away indignant. When he eventually did what he was told, he was healed of his leprosy.

  "Elisha sent a messenger to say to him, 'Go, wash yourself seven times in the Jordan, and your flesh will be restored and you will be cleansed.'" 2 King 5:10.

- This 'faith in action' occurred also when Jesus gave specific instructions to His disciples. When they did what Jesus said, there were occasions when miracles occurred. The feeding of the 5000 included directives to distribute five loaves of bread

and two fish. As this was done, the food multiplied.[1] When tax was due, Jesus instructed his disciples:
"...Go to the sea and cast a hook, and take the first
fish that comes up, and when you open its mouth
you will find a shekel; take that and give it to them
for me and for yourself" Matthew 17:27.

On a mission trip to Trinidad, we were allowed to speak to students in the public schools during their hour of religious instruction. We saw amazing miracles occurring that day. There was a young boy who was blind in his right eye who received his sight. There were numerous students asking for improved vision to be able to read the chalkboard. Over several minutes their vision cleared to be able to read easily. These were healthy students by and large, but there were healings of various simple aches and pains that provided a great demonstration of God's love for them and an opportunity for a response to the gospel. I learned when returning to the camp where we resided, a couple women on our team had stayed up all night in prayer. I am sure this is why we saw such great outpouring of God's Spirit that day.

One of the classrooms we attended had about eighty boys who were eleven and twelve years old. After a brief message, and while we were ministering healing to some of the boys, a few of them started pointing at a certain boy, saying, 'pray for his healing.' They were saying this in somewhat of a mocking tone. This boy suffered under the ridicule of his classmates because his face was crooked. The midline of his face from top to bottom was skewed to the right at his mandible. He had large front teeth that protruded forward from his mouth so much that he had trouble putting his lips together to cover his teeth.

I asked him if he wanted me to pray for him. The boys who were pointing at him continued to taunt him. He responded with a very slight nod. I think he was too wounded and insecure to speak. So I placed my hands on his jaw and commanded his face to straighten in the name of Jesus. I did not see any obvious change occurring, but maybe slightly. I asked him if he could feel something happening, but he did not answer me. So I told him to go to the boy's bathroom where there was a mirror and look for himself, then return to me. I was ministering to other boys when he returned about five minutes later. He simply did what he was told to do: go look at himself in the mirror and return. His face which was now straight and his teeth were in his mouth. The boys that were deriding him saw this, as well as the others in the class.

I heard from the youth director who led us to these various schools that there were 1800 boys in this public school. Over the next two or three days the teachers reported that there was peace and calm in the whole school. Everyone in the school knew about this boy because of the shape of his face. The word had spread about what had happened: this boy was healed by the touch of Jesus. Glory to God.

Other Means of Grace

There are other methods by which the Holy Spirit and His gifts were imparted to others. In the Old Testament it was common for the Holy Spirit's power to come upon kings, priests, and prophets through anointing with oil. Today some will use a small amount of olive oil on the tip of a finger when making the sign of a cross on the forehead of one receiving prayer.

A sacramental understanding of baptism recognizes this practice as a means by which God imparts his grace to people. There are many testimonies of newborn babies struggling to live who were baptized by a Pastor or a medical caregiver. Healing occurred through the water and the words of baptism. A sacramental understanding of the Lord's Supper or Holy Communion also recognizes it as a means of grace by which God strengthens and preserves a believer unto everlasting life.

Extraordinary Means

Jesus healed a blind man by spitting into the dirt to make mud and placing it over his eyes. He was then told to go and wash in the pool of Siloam.[2] At other times Jesus simply touched blind eyes to bring healing; He did not always use mud when restoring sight. Paul used a handkerchief to be brought to some people needing healing. And Peter's shadow, as it crossed over people near him, brought healing.

These extraordinary means indicate God's preference to heal through believers with a certain point of contact. Most commonly this was through the laying on of hands or touch. The focus is not on mud, handkerchiefs, or shadows, but on the presence of the Holy Spirit within believers making contact with people needing healing.

How To Begin

The above list shows biblical strategies for using the authority God gives to believers and releasing God's power for advancing His kingdom. Then how should one begin to use the authority bestowed by God in Christ?

I learned how to reduce a dislocated shoulder by first watching someone else who demonstrated and explained what needs to be done. Then when it was my turn, I copied what I saw and heard. There are many ways to reduce a dislocated shoulder, but I started by copying and reproducing what I was shown. Similarly when one learns to play guitar, the same process occurs where the student learns by watching first then doing just what he was shown. This is the same for almost any skill we might acquire. We do not gain such skills without actually repeatedly doing what is shown and taught.

This is a process of discipleship. The twelve disciples were with Jesus watching and learning from Him. Soon He sent them out to do the same things they observed Jesus doing. Then He commanded those disciples to make disciples of all nations, teaching them to observe what He had commanded them.

When Peter raised Tabitha from the dead, he did so by copying what he saw Jesus do when He raised a dead girl. Compare Jesus' account recorded in Luke 8 with how Peter copied what Jesus did as recorded in Acts 9.

> "While he was still speaking, a man from the ruler's house came and said, 'Your daughter is dead; do not trouble the Teacher any more.' But Jesus on hearing this answered him, 'Do not fear; only believe, and

she shall be well.' And when he came to the house, *he permitted no one to enter with him*, except Peter and John and James, and the father and mother of the child. And all were weeping and bewailing her; but he said, 'Do not weep; for she is not dead but sleeping.' And they laughed at him, knowing that she was dead. But taking her by the hand he called, saying, *'Child, arise.'* And her spirit returned, and she got up at once; and he directed that something should be given her to eat" Luke 8:49-56 (Italics mine).

"Now there was at Joppa a disciple named Tabitha, which means Dorcas. She was full of good works and acts of charity. In those days she fell sick and died; and when they had washed her, they laid her in an upper room. Since Lydda was near Joppa, the disciples, hearing that Peter was there, sent two men to him entreating him, 'Please come to us without delay.' So Peter rose and went with them. And when he had come, they took him to the upper room. All the widows stood beside him weeping, and showing tunics and other garments which Dorcas made while she was with them. *But Peter put them all outside* and knelt down and prayed; then *turning to the body he said, 'Tabitha, rise.'* And she opened her eyes, and when she saw Peter she sat up. And he gave her his hand and lifted her up. Then calling the saints and widows he presented her alive" Acts 9:36-41 (Italics mine).

It is a great blessing to know the general authority given to believers and the specific authority given to you, but this is only "book" knowledge until you use the authority you have been given. When you use the authority you have been given, then you gain more faith and knowledge of the mystery of this transcendent power residing in you. To use the authority given to you by God is to release the power of the Holy Spirit dwelling within you. The same power that raised Jesus from the dead dwells in believers. This power goes forth when you use your authority by speaking to this mountain, by touch and laying on of hands, and by putting faith in action.

Begin by doing and copying Jesus and His disciples as recorded in the Word of God. Begin by coming alongside those who are using their authority in order to observe and learn from them. Then go out and take some risks by doing the Word. Go to your family, to your friends, to co-workers, other believers in a church setting, and out to the marketplace. Get the Word of God into your heart. Get into a lonely place and pray. Then get into a public place and take risks. Use the authority you are given by God.

Chapter 28

Use Your Authority Wisely

I attended church regularly as I grew up, but the gospel message and a relationship with Jesus did not capture me until I saw some signs and wonders. Before this I do not know how many church services I attended and how many sermons I heard. I remember singing in the choir and the summer camps, but I cannot remember any of the messages delivered in the service or Sunday school classes. I do treasure the priority established by my parents to attend church regularly. Though there was no remarkable event or message that called me to live for Jesus, the investment of time in church with other believers was very important. I believed in God but did not think about it much. I thought God was distant and not directly active in His creation on earth. Before going away to college I did not ever see a demonstration of some ministry or circumstances that unquestionably called my attention to our Lord.

Then I attended a Holy Spirit conference in Wisconsin when I was eighteen years old. There I heard several prophecies that were given between some of the worship songs. At the time I did not know what was happening. I did not know about prophetic messages; nor did I pay much attention. Then a man approached the microphone and spoke in tongues. This got my attention as I knew no one could speak so distinctly and fluidly in an unlearned, different language without inspiration of the Holy Spirit. Now I was giving my full attention because a sign of God's presence was demonstrated. The leader then stated that we had been given a message in tongues and we should pray for interpretation. I remembered that this was a phenomenon that was reported in Scripture. I realized the God of history was active today and I wanted to hear what He would say, so I prayed for interpretation. Perhaps for the first time I was eager to hear the word of the Lord.

Another man then spoke words to interpret the unknown language. These words hit me. It was a message calling us to repent before it is too late and receive the cleansing blood of Jesus for salvation. Later in that same conference I watched an elderly woman with arthritis come to the front. The leader laid hands on her and ministered healing. She then bent over to touch her toes and jumped up and down without pain. These were demonstrations of the power and presence of God through gifts of the Holy Spirit manifested through regular, humble believers.

I had a seven hour drive back to the college I was attending. I had about seven hours of questions for the others traveling with me. They explained very well the basics of the gospel. I was struck with the truth that God loved me and that He was active in the world today. I was also aware that I needed to repent of my sins, ask forgiveness, and ask Jesus into my heart and life to become my Lord and Savior. Later that week while alone in my dormitory room I repented and committed my life to Jesus.

Holy Spirit Promptings

I am grateful for the individuals who boldly demonstrated the Holy Spirit and His power. Without these I would not likely have paid much attention or come to commit my life to Him. Because they obeyed the promptings of the Holy Spirit and used their gifts for the glory of God, I very quickly became aware that that God was active today, His words recorded in Scripture were relevant today, and He is worthy of my life commitment.

They were wise in their use of the gifts of the Holy Spirit. There were no antics or theatrics. There was no hype or excessive emotion. There was instead honesty and humility. They simply allowed the Holy Spirit to show Himself in a way that was acceptable to me and to most people. There was nothing weird or distasteful. No one spun around three times and spit on their shoulder in some effort to reproduce some strategy or method. There were no quirks or distractions that took me aside from the display of some of the glory of God. They used their authority wisely.

1 Corinthians 14:32 says "The spirits of prophets are subject to prophets." In other words, Spirit-filled believers can quench the indwelling Holy Spirit by neglect or disobedience — or these same believers can yield to the Holy Spirit by obedience to the Word of God and promptings of the Holy Spirit. God does not overrule our will and force us to do what He desires. When we do yield to the promptings of the Holy Spirit, we have freedom to express this in our own way, out of our own personality and vernacular. "The spirits of the prophets are subject to the prophets." Just as the Holy Spirit worked through Billy Graham in the Billy Graham way, so He will not bypass the personality and context of the individual in whom He dwells. He will work through your particular uniqueness. "All these are inspired by one and the same Spirit, who apportions to each one *individually* as he wills" 1 Corinthians 12:11 (Italics mine). When Spirit-filled believers wisely use their authority in Christ, there is an opportunity for the kingdom of God to be demonstrated.

There are many references in the Scriptures where God's people are led by the Spirit. Often the directives involved are very simple and brief. One example, recorded in Acts 8, is about Philip and the Ethiopian Eunich.

> "But an angel of the Lord said to Philip, 'Rise and go toward the south to the road that goes down from Jerusalem to Gaza.' This is a desert road. And he rose and went. And behold, and Ethiopian, a eunuch, a minister of the Candace, queen of the Ethiopians, in charge of all her treasure, had come to Jerusalem to worship and was returning; seated in his chariot, he was reading the prophet Isaiah. And the Spirit said to Philip, 'Go up and join this chariot.' So Philip ran to him, and heard him reading Isaiah the prophet, and asked, 'Do you understand what you are reading?'

And he said, 'How can I, unless someone guides me?'
And he invited Philip to come up and sit with him"
Acts 8:26-31.

Here the Spirit spoke briefly to Philip telling him to go south on the desert road toward Gaza. This was not Philip's original plan for that day. This meant Philip would leave his outreach team. Perhaps he could have questioned if he would have enough water and food to proceed on a desert road for an unknown distance. How would he rejoin the others with whom he was ministering? Despite these and maybe other potential consequences of going south toward Gaza, Philip obeyed what the Spirit told him. He obeyed without any further instructions or understanding why he should do this or what he would encounter. He simply proceeded south on the road to Gaza. As Philip obeyed this word, his faith and expectation was increased as he looked for further guidance from the Holy Spirit.

His simple obedience to a simple word placed him in position to hear one other brief, simple directive. As he went along the road he saw a man in a chariot. The Holy Spirit then spoke again for him to go over to that chariot. This was a very simple thing to do. When Philip obeyed the prompting of the Spirit, it became clear to him what divine appointment God had arranged. The Ethiopian Eunuch was reading from Isaiah. It was then obvious to Philip what to do and say as he explained the Scriptures to the Eunuch and led him to faith in Jesus Christ.

What has God told you to do? Do it then. Maybe He will not bring further revelation until you do what He told you earlier. Go back to the last prompting of the Holy Spirit that yet needs your response and obey it. Be faithful in little. Do the simple things. Follow the simple promptings.

This account of Philip's ministry to the Eunuch included two specific directives of the Holy Spirit. The rest of what happened apparently seemed clear enough to Philip. He saw the Eunuch reading the Scriptures and was prepared to answer questions and lead this man to faith in Jesus Christ. Most opportunities to minister to others occur without some initial prompting of the Holy Spirit. They occur as we go about our daily routines. Occasionally the Spirit of God will prompt us out of our regular activities, but we should not wait to minister to others until certain promptings or directives come. Rather we can look for such divine appointments as we go through each day. Some consider every encounter throughout any given day is a divine appointment. "For we are his workmanship, created in Christ Jesus for good works, which God prepared beforehand, that we should walk in them" Ephesians 2:10.

After finishing his ministry to the Ethiopian Eunuch, Philip was suddenly taken away by the Spirit and appeared next at Azotus where he continued to preach the Word of God on the way to Ceasarea. Azotus was about 25 miles from where Philip met with the Eunuch. This text seems to indicate Philip was transported by the Spirit. Amazing signs and wonders can occur with our ears tuned to the Holy Spirit and with simple obedience to Him.

Paul's Strategy

The church at Corinth was established by demonstrations of the power of the Holy Spirit. Just before coming to Corinth, Paul had been evangelizing in Athens where he tried to persuade people at the city center (Acts 17). There he used the inscription on the statue saying, "To an unknown God", to connect with some of the people, hoping to convince them by means of philosophical dialogue. Just a few people placed their faith in Jesus and others said they would like to hear more. Acts 18:1 says, "After this he [Paul] left Athens and went to Corinth." So Paul left Athens and arrived in Corinth. Then in his first letter to the Corinthians he stated what seems to be a shift in his strategy. The words "when I came to you brethren" show a contrast between persuasion evangelism and power evangelism.

> "When I came to you, brethren, I did not come pro-
> claiming the testimony of God in lofty words of
> wisdom, but in demonstration of the Spirit and of
> power. And I was with you in much weakness and
> trembling. And my speech and my message were not
> in plausible words of wisdom, but in demonstration
> of the power of the Holy Spirit, that your faith might

not rest in the wisdom of men, but in the power of
God" 1 Corinthians 2:1-5.

In Athens, Paul used persuasion and philosophical arguments to
advance the Gospel. At Corinth, Paul did not try to persuade people
with human wisdom. He simply proclaimed Jesus and Him crucified.
He also demonstrated the Holy Spirit and His power so that their faith
would not rest in the wisdom of men, but in the power of God. Later
in chapter 4, Paul says, "The Kingdom of God does not consist in
talk, but in power" 1 Corinthians 4:20.

A whole church was started by Paul's proclamation of Jesus
and His demonstrations of the Holy Spirit and of power. Prior to
this in Athens, only a few responded to Paul's persuasive attempts.
Furthermore, it seems that Paul was concerned that people might be
following his own wisdom rather than having faith in the power of
God. Paul used the authority given him by God to evangelize the
Corinthians. Compared to Athens, the results were great. There is
a time and place for persuasion evangelism, but our faith should
be centered in the power of God to save from sin, deliver from the
devil, heal diseases, and grant eternal life. Paul used power evangelism wisely to this end.

Compassion

Splanchnizomai (splagnizomai) is the Greek verb meaning 'to
have compassion' or 'to be moved in the inner parts.' It refers to
a yearning of the bowels, a deep gut feeling of concern for others.
There are anatomical structures in the abdomen that are named
after this Greek root: splanchnic circulation, splanchnic nerves, and
splanchnic mesoderm. Splanchnic refers to the viscera, the bowels.
Jesus had splanchnic compassion on the multitudes because they
were like sheep without a shepherd. He healed compassionately; He
healed people because He loved and cared for people.

His obedience to the Father brought Him to the cross to die for
our salvation and wholeness. This was the greatest act of love and
compassion. He laid down His authority and humbled Himself to
death on the cross. Therefore God has highly exalted Him above

every other authority.[1] He used His authority out of His compassion for people.

We can do the same. We should use our authority as believers as Jesus did. Wise use of authority comes out of attitudes of compassion. You will not always feel compassion for others, but we can always do acts of compassion regardless of our feelings at the time. We do not have to wait for compassionate feelings in order to use our authority in Christ to bless others. Those who act compassionately will sooner or later feel the compassion they are acting out.

Demonstration

Besides healing out of His compassion for people, Jesus also healed demonstratively. In addition to the blessing those healings were to the persons receiving it, these were signs and wonders that pointed to the presence of the kingdom of God and verified what Jesus taught. He did signs and wonders as a testimony to who He was and the truth of His words. Signs and wonders were not themselves to be the primary focus. They point to the Kingdom of God at hand and the great love of Jesus for people and for all creation. Jesus performed signs and wonders publically so people would see and believe in Him.

The disciples and apostles demonstrated the kingdom of God and used their authority in ways that did not call attention to themselves. Nevertheless, people were inclined to focus on those through whom God's power flowed. At times the onlookers attempted to worship them, but such self-glorification was refused and redirected to testify to the Lordship of Jesus Christ and bring glory to God.

Peter and John spoke to the onlookers after the paralytic was healed at the gate called Beautiful:

> "And when Peter saw it he addressed the people, 'Men of Israel, why do you wonder at this, or why do you stare at us, as though by our own power or piety we had made him walk?' ... And his name, by faith in his name, has made this man strong whom you see and know; and the faith which is through Jesus has given

the man this perfect health in the presence of you all"
Acts 3:12, 16.

The people on the island of Malta thought Paul was a god when he shook of a viper and had no ill effects.[2] A magician named Simon converted to faith in Jesus. He saw the demonstrations of the Holy Spirit, but then wanted to buy the power of the Holy Spirit from Philip. Peter rebuked him and called Simon's intentions a wickedness coming from a heart of bitterness and in bondage to iniquity. Simon repented of this agenda.[3]

So demonstrations of the Spirit and of the power of God brought many to place faith in Jesus Christ, but also brought some to misplace their worship, to seek the gift rather than the Giver, or to focus on the earthen human vessels rather than the transcendent power of God. People today are no different. Many come to faith in Jesus Christ through the preaching of the good news accompanied with signs and wonders, but very often believers in churches today identify certain few people who are associated with healing or other signs and wonders, not recognizing that healing is given to the whole church to minister one to another. Rather than having faith in God, they may place their faith in ones who have testified to and demonstrated healings and other displays of the Spirit's power. This places undo weight and temptation on these few who use their gifts and authority. This situation can be managed or averted by carefully giving glory to God, rejecting payment and position that some may offer, and by discipling others to wisely use their authority as believers so the whole body of Christ functions in their measure of faith and as the Holy Spirit apportions gifts.

Remember when Naaman the Syrian commander came with his army and many gifts to seek healing from Elisha. Elisha shied away from this fanfare and riches. He did not go himself to Naaman, but sent his servant Gehazi to bring his message instructing Naaman to wash seven times in the muddy Jordan River. Elisha did not place himself in a position where adulation and worldly things could derail his calling and ministry. Unfortunately Gehazi was overtaken by these offers from Naaman. He saw the riches and heard Naaman offer these gifts. As Naaman and his entourage were some distance away, Gehazi pursued them, falsely saying that Elisha did want the gifts offered.[4]

Manifestations

Despite the potential for misusing the gifts and authority given to us sinners, God still promises to show Himself to and through believers who love the Lord and obey Him. Here is a great promise from Jesus: "He who has my commandments and keeps them, he it is who loves me, and he who loves me will be loved by my Father, and I will manifest myself to him" John 14:21. When we are under God's authority and carefully obey His words, He will demonstrate and manifest himself to us. "To each is given the manifestation of the Spirit for the common good" 1 Corinthians 12:7. "For the eyes of the Lord run to and fro throughout the whole earth, to show his might on behalf of those whose heart is blameless toward him" 2 Chronicles 16:9.

Some of the greatest miracles I have seen occurred in a public setting, while other people were watching. It seems God is very willing to demonstrate Himself through the body of Christ. Such demonstrations are consistent with Scripture. I have come to prefer to minister healing with others watching as it seems that there is an increase of the number of people reporting improvement of symptoms from God's healing touch. This is the purpose of signs and wonders: to testify to the kingdom of God and the truth of His Word. First attempts to demonstrate the Holy Spirit and His power can feel like Peter possibly did when he stepped out of a boat to walk on water, but God honors this step of faith. In a church setting it can and should be quite normal and safe for believers to use their authority in Christ according to their measure of faith.

Time and Practice

To learn something involves time and practice. This is true also for the gifts of the Spirit and the ministry entrusted to the church. Such time and practice is the process of discipleship. Anyone who grows in authority does so by learning to know and use this authority.

Just as a soldier in the army learns and grows in leadership to eventually become a commander in a position of authority, so believers grow in authority by being faithful in little simple things. No army commander came into his position by performing perfectly every step along the way. Abundant grace and forgiveness exists for the believer learning to use authority wisely.

Servanthood

Jesus came to serve, not to be served. His intentions and actions were to serve and minister to others. Though He was the King of kings, He never used His authority or position to lord it over others. Jesus' life displayed servanthood. This attitude of service is part of Jesus' answer to the apostles when they asked Jesus to increase faith, as written in Luke 17. Here Jesus taught that the worker in the field at the end of a day of work does not expect to be served by his master. At the end of a day of work, the servant continues to serve his master, saying, "We are unworthy servants. We have only done our duty." This servanthood was Jesus' attitude and actions. His answer to the apostles' request for increased faith included this same attitude of service and obedience. Faith is increased by doing your duty in an attitude of service.

Selfless

The authority given to believers is not for selfish goals or ambition. According to James 3:16: "Where selfish ambition and bitter jealousy exist, there will be disorder and every vile practice." Selflessness or death to self is an essential, foundational requirement for disciples of Jesus. He said to all, "If any man would come after me, let him deny himself and take up his cross daily and follow me" Luke 9:23. Part of the necessary preparations for ministering healing to others involves a reminder of being dead to self and alive to God in Christ Jesus.

Pray for the mind of Christ and a desire to do His will, setting aside any personal desires that may be selfish. As we abide in Him, His Spirit works in us to help us to want what He wants, to make His desires our own desires. "For God is at work in you, both to will and to work for his good pleasure" Philippians 1:6. "And this then is the confidence we have in him, that when we abide in him and he in us, we can ask whatever we desire and it will be done" John 15:7.

Know and Use Your Authority

Get the Word into your heart. Get into a private place and pray. Get into a public place and take risks. Do the Word. Know and use your God given authority for advancing God's kingdom. This is the faith of the Centurion. This is the mustard seed faith that can move THIS MOUNTAIN from here to there.

"A compelling first-hand experience of the fascinating world of neuropsychiatry. Witnessing this master clinician at work fuels a realistic optimism about recovery from even the most extreme afflictions of the mind."

Michael Norden MD, Psychiatrist.
University of Washington, Seattle.
Author of the important related text, "Beyond Prozac".

"Cry the Beloved Mind fascinates and educates. The reader is allowed insights into major discoveries through dramatic explorations of medical information interspersed with social issues. A remarkable contribution, you should not do without."

Melvin Morse, MD, Pediatrician.
Author of the best seller, "Closer to the Light".

"This book takes us on a voyage to the most mysterious destination of all, the human mind. Vernon Neppe is a wonderful guide. Using the Socratic method practiced by all great teachers, Dr. Neppe takes us into the clinic with patients where we all join him on his daily exploration of discovery and hope."

Paul Perry, Arizona.
Many times New York Times Best-selling Author.

"More than a mere book, this is a voyage that can help thousands of lost souls with the awareness that given detailed evaluations, modern medicine can help even the most difficult of brain conditions."

Jay Luxenberg MD.
Internist, University of California, San Francisco.
Author of "Residential Care".

i